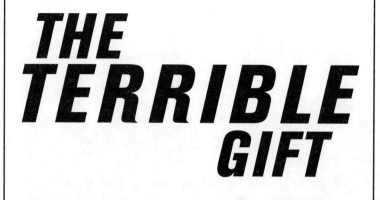

THE TERRIBLE GIFT

The Brave New World of
GENETIC MEDICINE

RICK J. CARLSON

GARY STIMELING

PUBLICAFFAIRS

New York

Book design by Jane Raese

Library of Congress Cataloging-in-Publication data
Carlson, Rick J.
The terrible gift: the brave new world of genetic medicine /
Rick J. Carlson, Gary Stimeling.—1st ed.
p. cm.
Includes bibliographical references and index.
ISBN 1-891620-65-7 (hbk.)
1. Medical genetics—Social aspects. I. Stimeling, Gary. II. Title
RB155.C375 2002
616180180180'.042—DC21
2001030392

FIRST EDITION

10 9 8 7 6 5 4 3 2 1

To my children–Becca, Josh, Blue, and Joey–
who have all wondered what I do, and may now understand
more about what's important,
even if they still won't know what I do.

–R. J. C.

To my beloved wife, Maureen,
and to our beloved cat, Mora,
whose familiar presence on my desk kept me going
through the project's end, and hers.

–G. S.

We have corrected Thy work and founded it upon

miracle, mystery and *authority*. And men rejoiced that

they were again led like sheep, and that the terrible gift

that brought them such suffering was, at last,

lifted from their hearts.

–The Grand Inquisitor
speaking to Jesus in Dostoyevsky's
The Brothers Karamazov (Book V, Chapter 5),
translated by Constance Garnett

Contents

Acknowledgments

Among numerous others, we would especially like to thank: Josh Carlson, researcher extraordinaire (Oh, the energy of the young!); our editors, Karl Weber and Paul Golob, for keeping us on track; our copy editor, Kate Scott, for helpful suggestions too numerous to count; Maureen Sugden, the Graig Nettles of copy editors, for unpaid work as a final pair of eyes; our publisher, Peter Osnos, and our agent, Peter Matson, for believing in the project from the beginning; and, for invaluable feedback and criticism, Ryan Phelan of Direct Medical Knowledge, Savary and Christine Phaeton (friends in deed), Clem Bezold of the Institute for Alternative Futures, Wendy Everett and Geoff Nilsen of the Institute for the Future, Sabeth Ireland, Paul Glynn, Charlie Smith, and Florence Comite.

Preface

The initial impetus for writing this book was to assess the effects that genetic science will have on our health-care system. But as we dove into the deep waters—the implications that arise from mapping the human genome in particular and from biotechnology in general—we soon realized that the book would have to encompass more than the health-care system itself. It would have to address the sweeping changes in all our lives that will result from biotechnology.

It's a bracing challenge. The new knowledge will profoundly transform the way we think and the way we live, much as the theory of evolution changed our sense of our place in nature and much as computers and the Internet are altering our daily activities.

However, genomics *will* revolutionize health care, perhaps faster and more thoroughly than it will affect the rest of society. Naturally, then, we concentrate on medicine as we discuss the gifts of genomics and their terrible implications. We do so not only because health care will experience such great changes but also because that field will encounter the most difficult economic, social, and moral conflicts. Health care will be on the leading edge in the struggle to extract real human value from the discoveries to come.

We now spend almost one fifth of our entire gross domestic product on health care. The life- and health-enhancing advances emerging from the laboratories could raise that proportion to one fourth, or even one third—if they are merely poured into the tin cup of our current system. Genomic medicine may well demonstrate a kind of "reverse alchemy"—not gold from dross but rather the gold of new technologies transformed into the base metal of inefficient, overpriced, unjust medicine.

Genomics will force us to decide what we are willing to pay for health care, in costs both financial and social. Because of its size and power, our health-care system might be compared to a mighty river. As therapeutic medicine expands and entirely new currents of upgrade medicine improve human endowments and performance, that stream could overflow its banks and inundate all other aspects of life. The flood will be hard to resist, for the new medicine will seduce us with the promise of longer life and easy ways to grasp the phantom called happiness.

Collectively Americans seem to believe that every problem has a technological fix, so we always use medicine, in part, to remedy what we've done to ourselves. We made that decision many decades ago when we built a curative health-care system rather than a preventive one. As we charted the river of health care, we built our settlements downstream where multitudes in need of repair would land on our banks, instead of upstream where the sources of our pathologies could be more easily diverted. The central irony about genetic medicine is that it is inherently preventive and thus a poor fit for our delivery system.

This book is an aggressive, in-your-face look at what we must do to reap the benefits of biotechnological medicine. If we have the collective will to redesign our health-care system in preparation for genomics, we will thereby escape from the cul-de-sac that our current setup has driven us into—a dead-end of intolerable costs for a product of ever-declining value in terms of the health it yields.

Parts of the text may rub some health-care managers and opinion leaders the wrong way. But the job ahead is too important to leave to the easily offended. Argue with us if you wish; point out our excesses of enthusiasm or cynicism. But if the ideal of a truly fair and powerful medicine appeals to you, please look beyond the faults in our argument and toward the common goal of enduring, beneficial change. That's what we've tried to do—engage readers in thinking and acting to create a better future.

Introduction

January 7, 2009—A schoolteacher in Hoboken, New Jersey, calls in sick. Janet McCarthy's bones ache. Every joint in her body gives her a shooting pain at the slightest movement. Thinking she has a new strain of the flu, she takes to her bed and doses herself with aspirin, chicken soup, and herbal teas. Her third-graders ply her with crayoned get-well cards.

After five days, the convulsions start. Friends check Janet into the local hospital, where the staff are baffled and increasingly frightened. She is vomiting and has severe diarrhea. The bones in her arms and legs have become soft, almost rubbery. Her skin feels as though it's on fire, and she becomes delirious. Her doctors try numerous drugs, but none of them work.

In three weeks, Janet is dead.

Meanwhile, fourteen of her twenty-four students and five of her colleagues at East Hudson Day School have developed similar symptoms and are rapidly traveling down the same terminal road. Physicians are unable to do more than alleviate their pain somewhat. Quickly realizing that they are dealing with a new contagious disease, public health authorities quarantine the town, then all of Hudson County, but to no avail. Soon, more than a dozen cities in the United States and England report new cases. However, investigators find no evidence of contact among victims of the early outbreaks. By the end of March, nearly every hospital in North America and Europe has at least a few cases. Many hospitals have four or five times more patients than they can possibly handle, and still the victims keep coming.

Throughout the spring, as increasing numbers of people succumb to the deadly disease, panic spreads, and most commercial activity grinds to a halt. The President of the United States directs the armed forces to take over sanitation and food distribution, but by midsummer there are too many casualties. Soon the President himself is dead, and the relief effort dissolves into chaos.

Meanwhile, biologists work around the clock to solve the mystery of the epidemic, which has come to be known as torturant plague or, more simply, "the death." It has an incubation period of five to six months, during which it is highly contagious via exhaled air, contaminated surfaces, or sexual contact. As a result, it has already spread widely before symptoms appeared in the first cases. Researchers believe that it was released in the late summer of 2008. They trace it as far as a factory in Nutley, New Jersey, that makes glue used on envelopes and stamps throughout the world. This glue, it now appears, has served as the initial vector, or carrier, to disseminate the pathogen invisibly. As their first project of the school year, Ms. McCarthy's class had sent letters to congressional leaders thanking them for passing the School Renovation Act.

Scientists never find out who made the germ. Charting the course of the infection in the human body turns out to be the last achievement of Western medical science.

The plague is caused by a new type of organism, a synthetic hybrid soon named *Bacillovirus clandestinus.* It is cunningly designed for maximum stealth and lethality, genetically engineered with resistance to all known antibiotics. It consists of a bacterium that carries within it a retrovirus similar to HIV. A retrovirus takes control of the cell it infects by inserting its own genetic material into the host cell's DNA. The bacterium and virus have been designed to protect each other from the immune system. The renegade scientists who created the plague have done so by adapting the technique that nearly eliminated malaria a few years ago. The surgeon general comments, "It is horribly ironic that one of medicine's greatest triumphs has been perverted to become our worst medical disaster."

In response to the anthrax attack of 2001 and other bioterrorism episodes, biologists learned to create drugs for new diseases more quickly. However, the composite nature of this organism and its long incubation period work against researchers, and the epidemic claims slightly more than 1 billion lives in 2009. Many cities of North America, Europe, and the Pacific Rim are completely wiped out by autumn. The contagion spreads more slowly into South America, Africa, India, China, and central Asia, and strict quarantines in these areas seem to be preserving some rural populations in medieval isolation. Thus there is some hope that humanity may survive, even if modern civilization does not.

XXXX

Doctors make the best killers. Their detailed knowledge of the human body gives them unique leverage for causing pain and death. Many historians and forensic specialists suspect that Jack the Ripper was a surgeon. New Jersey's infamous "Doctor X" murdered at least 20 patients with curare, a poison derived from a tree of the Amazon jungle, in the late 1960s. Beginning in 1985, Michael Swango, the "Doctor of Death," is believed to have killed as many as 60 patients in the United States and Zimbabwe. With institutional support, the Nazi physician Josef Mengele achieved far more prodigious numbers. Today Osama bin Laden's henchman Ayman al-Zawahiri, an Egyptian specialist in the genital mutilation of girls for religious purposes and the man who plotted the assassination of Anwar al-Sadat, seeks to outdo even Mengele by carrying out terrorist attacks using chemical and biological weapons.

In the past, such men, so atypical of their profession, have had power only as far as their hands could reach, or as small cogs in a much larger machine of destruction. Now biotechnology will give them enormous power, power that we only dimly understand. Indeed, mistakes by the well-intentioned could do almost as much damage as the worst-case scenario outlined above. And treatments that are entirely beneficial to individuals may have far-reaching negative effects on society and the natural world. New medical technologies are being developed in thousands of industrial and scientific facilities around the globe, sometimes with rigorous controls, sometimes not. Under the pressure of competition, for-profit companies have every incentive to rush new products to market. Will they all be safe? Will some have unpredictable side effects? No one can say. The only thing we know for sure is that unprecedented powers are emerging whose full impact is impossible to predict.

This book deals with the medical breakthroughs of tomorrow—their promise and their peril. We emphasize the peril, not because we believe that the new medicine will be altogether destructive but because too little attention is being paid to the dangers it poses.

Medicine's New Role

As it unravels the secrets of life, medicine itself is undergoing unparalleled changes. The profession has only recently been transformed into a commercial industry. Now another reorientation is beginning. A new, immensely profitable, consumer-oriented medicine is emerging.

In the past, doctors aspired to cure the sick and hoped only to do a better job of it someday. Now suddenly they can foresee comprehensive therapies for almost all diseases. But that's only the beginning. Armed with our emerging scientific understanding of the chemistry of life, medicine will go far beyond the traditional role of curing and into the realm of making people stronger, smarter, and sexier. Doctors are developing the ability to improve our lives in dozens of other ways. They expect to be able to amend all facets of life—mood, energy, alertness, productivity, endurance, sexual response, appearance, intelligence, strength, the acuity of the senses, the experience of pleasure—according to their clients' taste, and not just temporarily but permanently.

To some degree, of course, medicine always has catered to the desire to be better, as opposed to merely not sick. The rich and powerful have had perennial access to such measures, often above the law. Soon after testosterone and growth hormones were discovered in the 1920s, manly millionaires were going to the Bahamas to be injected with extracts of ram testes and sheep embryos. John F. Kennedy had his amphetamines and steroid "vi-

5

tamin" shots from Max Jacobson, better known as "Dr. Feel-good." Richard Nixon reportedly experimented with a private supply of Dilantin to control his paranoia and mood swings at a time when the drug was not available to the public.

Now, however, our ingenuity is about to bring a huge new wave of such improvements to, if not the masses, at least the upper and maybe the middle classes. This wave will vastly expand the traditional boundaries of what we thought medicine could or should do, whether by means of public or private financing.

These innovations will be startling and in many ways wonderful. They will make people stronger, smarter, and more resistant to illness, or just different, with blue eyes instead of brown, clear skin instead of freckled, fast-twitch (sprinter's) muscle fibers instead of slow-twitch (distance-runner's). Our genetic operating systems will become as upgradable as computer software, and perhaps as reliable.

There's no denying the appeal of the new medical vision. At one time or another, we've all wished we could revise our physical and mental endowments. But these medical advances are coming at us so quickly that we are groping for context, a framework in which to think clearly, as responsible citizens of the earth, about the pros and cons of our new powers before we're swept away by them.

One thing seems certain: Much of the dream will be expensive, in both dollars and sense. More and more, the medicine of the future will address itself to those with money to spend on remodeling. It will become a potent force pitting class against class. It will raise thorny questions about payment, fair access, and responsible use. The answers we come up with will help determine what kind of society we'll have in the twenty-first century.

Biotechnology promises ultimate power over life itself. As one of biotechnology's key delivery channels, medicine will help determine the new industry's value in human terms. This new medical science will truly be a *terrible* gift–terrible in its ability to inspire dread and awe. It promises new freedoms–notably freedom from disease and the freedom to change genetic traits that until now have been fixed for life. But it also will bring us fearsome new dangers and responsibilities. And if we are to cope with these burdens, we must first understand them.

PART ONE

The Medical-Industrial Complex

C H A P T E R   1

The Advent of Genetic Medicine

TOMORROW'S MEDICINE WILL HAVE amazing new powers, and breakthrough treatments are coming faster than most people realize. Already genetic therapy can cure severe combined immune deficiency (SCID), a disease that heretofore meant swift and certain death for any infant born with it. To understand such innovative cures, a basic knowledge of the underlying science is essential. In this chapter, we'll provide an overview

— relatively straight forward, easy.
— very rare

of the scientific basics you need to know in order to grasp the implications of genetic medicine. Then we'll offer a quick tour of one of the most immediately promising research arenas—drug design. Our goal is to make clear how vast the possibilities of medical research are for both good and evil.

Biology, the study of life and its self-written instruction book, has given rise to biotechnology, our nascent ability to write instructions of our own, combining old life forms to create new life forms as varied as the stories we make with words made from letters. Biotechnology now begins to gather unto itself several previously independent foundations of human society—agriculture, wildlife management and animal husbandry, food preparation, manufacturing, and medicine. Our first reading of the human genetic code combines with advances in materials science and information technology to change everything—for the better, we all hope.

Most of what you need to know about molecular genetics in order to follow the discussion in the rest of this book is presented here:

Two slightly acidic chemicals—DNA (deoxyribonucleic acid) and RNA (ribonucleic acid)—are found in the nucleus of every cell. Together they convey genetic information. Long chains of DNA store the genetic information. Short lengths of RNA transcribe and communicate segments of the genetic code as needed to other parts of the cell. DNA is sometimes compared to a master blueprint, while RNA serves as the working drawings for various parts of the building.

The structure of the DNA molecule is like a ladder. This ladder is enormously long, and its two stringers, or side struts, spiral about each other in the familiar double helix pattern.

A single unit of this ladder, consisting of a piece of one of the stringers and half of a rung, is called a *nucleotide*. Each nucleotide is composed of three molecular subunits: a sugar, a phosphate group, and a specialized information-carrying subunit called a *base*. The sugars and phosphates line up lengthwise to make the stringers. There are four bases—adenine, thymine, cytosine, and guanine—and these combine in pairs to form the rungs. Thus each base is linked to its own portion of stringer and to another base.

These *base-pairs* always form in the same combinations: adenine and thymine (AT or TA), and cytosine and guanine (CG or GC). In other words, the genetic code can be thought of as a language written with an alphabet that has only four "letters," each of which is symbolized by two letters of the Roman alphabet: AT, TA, CG, and GC. It is the sequence of these base-pairs that encodes genetic information. A fifth base, uracil, replaces thymine in RNA, but in other respects RNA encodes information in the same way as DNA.

Properly speaking, "nucleotide" refers to a unit of the DNA molecule's *structure*, while "base-pair" refers to its unit of *information*. In practice, this amounts to the same thing, and, to prevent confusion, please note that the two terms are often used interchangeably.

Adjacent nucleotides are grouped in different permutations of three, called *codons*. In the genetic language, each codon denotes an amino acid, one of the 20 molecular Legos of which the proteins that build every component of every living thing on earth are constructed. Groups of three are needed to spell out the 20 amino acid "words" using only four base-pair "letters."

A *gene* is a part of the DNA molecule that contains complete instructions for building one protein or for a modifying action performed by one gene upon others. In general, it takes at least

20,000 base-pairs to make a gene; some genes require as many as 100,000, or even more. Thousands of genes in turn are grouped together to form a *chromosome,* which is actually one enormous DNA molecule millions of nucleotides long. To continue the language analogy, a gene might be considered a "sentence" or a "paragraph," a complete unit of thought, while a chromosome is like a "chapter" in the book of life that describes a particular species. The correspondence is not exact, of course, since language is not the same as life. For example, genes seem to be arranged, both within each chromosome and among all of a species' chromosomes, by the happenstance of evolution rather than according to any logical design.

In order to synthesize protein, information must be gotten out of the gene and taken to the place where the new protein is to be made. To understand how this is accomplished, we're going to have to switch metaphors slightly. Imagine a ladder that can be split down the middle of its rungs, kind of like a zipper. Then imagine half of another zipper that slips in to temporarily fit against one exposed side of this portion of the DNA molecule. This is much like what happens to portions of the DNA molecule when a single gene within it is *activated* and then "read" by a length of RNA. Actually there are several forms of RNA and several helper enzymes involved in the activation, transcription, and transfer of genetic information, but to describe them all would take us into a level of scientific detail that is not needed for our purposes.

The "one gene, one protein" system we have summarized here has itself turned out to be simpler than the facts of nature. Most genes actually consist of modules, called *exons*, which can be combined in various orders. Many exons can even function as parts of several different genes. The exons are separated by long stretches of extraneous material, called *introns*, which are not part of any gene. It is as though the genes were a deck of playing cards shuffled into a huge stack of jokers.

To make a certain protein, RNA copies out the required exons. These "cards" are then combined into a "hand" in a cellular assembly system called a *spiceosome*, where the protein synthesis takes place. Most genes contribute to making many different proteins, depending on the number and order of exons used. In every cell of our bodies, various exons of various genes are constantly being activated and copied out to produce the proteins needed to keep our cells functioning.

Most genes contribute to making many different proteins, depending on the number and order of exons used. Only a small fraction of the total complement of genes is in use at a given time in a given cell type, and, taken together, all of the genes constitute only a small fraction of our DNA, 1 or 2 percent. The non-genetic DNA, primarily the introns, includes some codes that boost or dampen the expression of nearby genes, but most of it seems defunct, a collection of deactivated viruses, bad first drafts, backup copies of working genes, spare parts for future genes, and filler. Evolution seems to keep its front yard littered with junk cars, rusted-out washing machines, and piles of old newspapers.

Genetics is the study of individual genes. *Genomics* is the study of an organism's genome, its complete set of genes. Aspects of genetics and genomics have given rise to new branches of learning. One example is the study of *single nucleotide polymorphisms*, or SNPs (pronounced "snips"). A SNP is a base-pair location in the gene at which any one of two or more different base-pairs may occur in a given individual. It's a variant spelling, like the difference between "spake" and "spoke." SNPs are the source of most physical differences between individuals of the same species. From the study of SNPs–SNPology, if you will–arises the emergent craft of tailoring medicines to a person's idiosyncratic array of SNPs, called *pharmacogenomics*.

Working outward from the level of the gene, the proteome is an organism's total complement of proteins. *Proteomics*–also called structural genomics–is the study of the human proteome, the estimated 100,000 proteins–each one synthesized in various cells from the chemical recipes in genes–that together make up our entire structure and metabolism. If the genome is the source code, the proteome is the shrink-wrapped software.

At the summit of this tower of learning and research is *genetic therapy*, the ability to edit the human book of life. With it we seek the ability to delete disease. Then we hope to go further, to search the cellular text for dull words and replace them with ones that sparkle.

This book is not about medicine's technological particulars, however. The concepts presented here should enable you to understand the discussions that follow. We'll present additional scientific detail only as needed. We're more concerned with the shape and outcome of new biological knowledge, and with how it will affect medicine's abilities and social role.

Drug Making from the Genes Up

One of the first fields of medicine to be revolutionized by genetics will be pharmacology. Genetic databases are computerized repositories of information about the base-pair sequence and the physiological function of genes. They are still in their infancy, but already they are giving birth to the next generation of drug design. Traditionally, to develop a new drug, pharmacologists would test an array of compounds for action on a target protein. The new pharmacology works in the reverse of the traditional way. Instead, drug chemists are looking for genes and proteins that seem amenable to manipulation by compounds they have in hand. For example, Incyte is a company that has compiled and sells access to a database much like a "selected bibliography" of genes with probable medical usefulness. Working from a gene in this database, researchers at Johnson & Johnson found a new histamine receptor in the thalamus of the brain. It is responsible for drowsiness caused by antihistamines, and knowledge of it should lead to the development of new antihistamines that don't make you sleepy, and also to new wakefulness drugs.

New techniques of nongenetic biological analysis are also playing a role in the synthesis of new drugs. Three-dimensional computer visualization and stereotactic mapping (pinpointing cell components down to the molecular level with regard to a reference grid) have been applied to drug synthesis for over a decade. So far the results from these two techniques have been disappointing, except for a few isolated successes like the AIDS drug Viracept, an advance in treatment–though not a cure–for AIDS.

Dissimilarities among patients mean that even if a drug gets to the right receptors on the right cells, in some people it will work but in others it will be ineffective, perhaps even harmful. The osteoarthritis drug Celebrex is an example of the uncertainty that biochemical idiosyncrasies of individual human organisms have on traditional drug design.

During its development, Celebrex (the generic name is celecoxib) looked like the first truly safe and effective drug to treat the pain of osteoarthritis. It works by inhibiting release of prostaglandins, messenger chemicals that can make pain-sensing neurons overreactive. Aspirin works the same way, but Celebrex inhibits a recently discovered class called cox-2 prostaglandins, which are produced *only* by inflamed tissue, leaving the others, made by healthy cells, alone. As a result, it seemed orders of magnitude better at relieving osteoarthritis pain than any previous drug, with very few adverse effects in over two years of testing on 13,000 people. Most important, it does not cause the bleeding stomach ulcers that result from heavy use of ibuprofen and naproxen. The most common "side effects" were beneficial ones—improvement of Alzheimer's disease and prevention of colon cancer.

Well, that was the clinical trials. In practice, the full spectrum of patients proved more diverse than even the unusually large number on whom the drug was tested. After more than three years of use, doctors have found that, although Celebrex represents an improvement, its benefits to many patients aren't as dramatic as expected, especially considering that it costs ten times as much as older drugs.

Still, advertising raised expectations and created a huge demand. The drug has a potential therapeutic market of some 40 million Americans. It was developed by a partnership between Searle (owned by Monsanto) and Pfizer and was released in February 1999. Celebrex and Merck's similar Vioxx together reaped $2 billion in their first year. Celebrex drove Pfizer's income for 1999 well above even its Viagra returns of the year before. That proves the demand, but Celebrex now seems like a step on the road to satisfying it, rather than the journey's much-desired destination.

The widely varying responses to drugs are due to a number of factors—differences in weight, nutrition, health, and levels of environmental toxins—but largely they result from SNPs. Out of 3.12

billion base-pairs in the human genome, about 99.8 percent are identical in all people. Nearly all of our nonmutational genetic differences reside in the other 0.2 percent.

Most of these 6 million or so SNPs are probably irrelevant to our physiology, since they occur outside genes, in the so-called junk DNA. But an estimated 300,000 to 700,000 of them occur in functional genes in 1 percent of the population or more, which is often enough to be considered medically significant. These relatively few SNPs are the primary determinants of human vulnerability to multifactorial, partly genetic diseases like cancer, asthma, and arteriosclerosis, as well as our varied reactions to drugs and environmental poisons.

In April 1999, 10 pharmaceutical companies and five nonprofit research institutions joined the Wellcome Trust of London, the world's largest medical philanthropy, to launch an effort to catalogue most of the important human SNPs by the end of 2001. The National Institute of Environmental Health Sciences is funding the Environmental Genome Project to study SNPs in relation to pollutants, and at least four companies are compiling their own SNP databases for sale by subscription to drug researchers.

SNP databases will not produce their full quota of medical advances directly. They will be like maps consisting only of contour lines and the shapes of rivers and shorelines, without labels. Others must then annotate the SNPs, that is, figure out what the variations in the proteins mean to the body, identifying those involved in specific diseases and modifiable with specific chemicals.

SNP mapping will bear most of its therapeutic fruit when combined with the rapidly maturing technology of genomic profiling, which allows doctors and researchers to observe gene activity in specific cells. This technology, also called *tissue transcript profiling* or *expression profiling,* uses microarray assay chips, glass slides on which thousands of microscopic dots of various RNA sequences have been placed. Activated genes in a sample solution that is washed over the chip react with the dots of RNA. Dyes or other chemical markers incorporated into the RNA dots change during the reaction, providing a comprehensive picture of gene activation in the tissue from which the sample solution was prepared.

The first generation of these chips has entered commercial use for testing small groups of genes, and a second generation is emerging for more complete analyses. These chips show which genes are active (that is, they are making proteins), for example, in neurons compared to muscle cells, or in one type of cancer compared to another type and to healthy tissue.

The large cancer-treatment centers have become the first users of such chips. The knowledge the chips afford is beginning to let oncologists choose drugs matched to the biochemical specifics of a patient's tumor, for maximum results with minimum time wasted on chemicals that turn out to be toxic or ineffective. Doctors have found, for example, that whereas several chemotherapeutics are highly poisonous to persons who lack a deactivation enzyme called thiopurine methyltransferase, the same drugs can be used in them effectively at a tenth or twentieth of the usual dose.

During the next decade, genomic assay methods will grow in speed, power, and affordability. Soon scientists will be able to compare the entire genomes of people prone to hypertension to those of people resistant to it, those of people who respond to Prozac to those of people who don't. Then they will be able to focus their studies on the SNPs involved. At present, some two dozen companies are hard at work on at least six dozen genechip techniques and product lines in a field that will be among the hottest of a hot industry in the current decade.

Reading the Body One Molecule at a Time

That's still only the beginning. The human genome sequence has yielded well over 10,000 genes whose proteins are "exported" from the cells in which they're made and thus are thought to be potential targets for drugs whose potency will lie in their ability to affect the "trade routes." However, the functions of most of those extracellular proteins are still unknown. Therefore, numerous companies and research institutes around the world are starting to collaborate on the goal of developing ways to take an inventory of all of the proteins in a tissue sample or an organism.

The problems are more complex than those encountered in sequencing a genome. Each protein has its own structure and composition, often involving thousands of amino acids and hundreds of thousands of atoms. Most proteins can assume various three-dimensional shapes and folding patterns, each producing a different chemical activity. (For example, badly folded proteins called prions are thought to cause mad-cow disease.) Different proteins can have the same or overlapping metabolic functions. In addition, human cells often modify standard-issue proteins by adding small molecular subunits not called for in the genetic instructions.

With current methods, it may take months to determine the shape and architecture of one protein. Any useful proteome sequencing method must do at least a hundred per hour. All this information must be correlated to gene transcription on the one hand, and to cell and body function on the other, in terms of both process (chemical reactions) and molecular structure—and in both health and disease. Finally, to be useful in drug design, all this knowledge has to be integrated into computer models of metabolism. This new biological mapping science is called *bioinformatics,* which can be thought of as a kind of computer-aided design system for the human body.

Along with the details of genetics and metabolism, computerized bioinformatics models also store information on drug chemistry and millions of previous drug tests, so as to predict how new compounds might act and to allow testers to profit from experience with related chemicals instead of reinventing the wheel each time. Software then compares the possible molecules with ones previously studied, discarding all that are obviously inert, carcinogenic, or laden with side effects. Thus researchers seeking a drug for a particular job can screen 50 million potential compounds in a day or two. Only the top few dozen candidates need be studied further.

Now 3D animation of molecular interactions comes into play. Researchers can do preliminary tests via computer simulations— *"in silico."* Simulations can cheaply weed out potential products that otherwise would fail in the first or second round of tests. Then, to get the most out of trials on animals and humans, programs can factor in variations of size and metabolism to set dosages, and even allow for patients' forgetting to take their pills. These simulations greatly decrease lab costs and shorten the lead time for getting FDA approval to market the drug.

During the next decade, biologists will complete their interlinked computer models of the entire human metabolism down to the molecular level. Drug makers will pretest their wares on virtual patients with ever greater reliability. They'll be able to ask, "If I have a compound that deactivates such and such an enzyme while increasing the supply of peptide X and hormone Y, how will it affect the immune system's response to HIV infection?"— and they'll get a testable answer from the computer.

That's when the most rewarding diagnostic and curative work will begin. Whole-genome assays of individual patients will quickly screen for hundreds of potentially disease-abetting weaknesses. Today, early proteome chips can already show simple reactions to 10,000 microdots of individual proteins on a glass microscope slide. With later versions, pharmacologists will be able to test a possible drug against all the enzymes and structural proteins in, say, melanoma cells or brain cells damaged by Alzheimer's. Then pharmacogenomics, the "output side" of this technology, will let chemists build each drug in an array of slightly different forms, helping doctors at last reach their age-old goal of being able to prescribe "the right drug at the right dose in the right patient at the right time."

At least half a dozen companies are working on chips to test the genes of AIDS patients and other chips to track strains of the fast-mutating AIDS virus itself, in hopes of predicting which of the currently available drugs will work best in each case. Though it's still in a very early stage, the effort has yielded a 10 percent improvement in the condition of the test groups over control groups in some studies. In a few years, SNP and proteome evaluation will become standard procedure before most treatments.

Genetic Therapy at the Threshold

In 1998, a medical milestone more important than the development of Viagra was reached—with considerably less fanfare. Doctors achieved the first successful genetic therapy in humans. In other words, they began using the human genetic code directly in pursuit of medical goals.

Several teams of cardiologists in Boston, New York, and Dallas have successfully treated some of their most severely ill heart-disease patients with genetic medicine. They've been injecting the gene for vascular endothelial growth factor (VEGF) directly into the heart muscle. The gene grew a network of new blood vessels, giving most of the damaged hearts and their owners a new lease on life. Angina pain was dramatically reduced or eliminated. True, the new coronary arteries were tiny, but no one had expected it to be so easy to get any results at all.

These experimenters used naked DNA, copies of the gene alone, with no *vector,* or carrier, such as a modified virus or other biological transport system, to carry it into the cells. Other researchers had just found that naked-DNA injections of a different gene could restore muscle tone in old mice. These experiments have proved that the proper genes, injected like any other drug, can help reverse some degenerative diseases, even before we understand all the intricacies of tissue growth.

If DNA injection were to enter standard practice only for heart disease, and only as a buyer of time rather than a cure, it would yield great savings in life, pain, and money. If further tests go as well as the early ones, this interim technique might replace or postpone much cardiac bypass surgery and angioplasty, which in any case fail a third or half the time. This new treatment could become standard practice as soon as 2002.

At present, however, routine genetic therapy in humans must still clear several high hurdles. It is possible with current techniques to replace specific defective genes in certain human cells in vitro (i.e., in the lab, not in the body), but the process is very inefficient. Only a few out of millions of target cells incorporate the gene into their DNA. Generally it gets absorbed at a random position. Some genes depend on adjacent triggers and other position cues, so preexisting genes and/or the new genes may not work right if the new DNA is absorbed at the wrong position.

Cells that do incorporate a working gene must then be cultured to at least 20 cell divisions for doctors to have enough to work with. A cell cannot go on dividing indefinitely; eventually a *cell line*, or series of daughter cells, becomes senescent, usually after about 50 divisions. (This limit is called the Hayflick limit, after its discoverer, the biologist Leonard Hayflick.) Genetic modifications must be made one at a time and the successfully modified cells must be isolated and cultured each time. Hence, the significance of the Hayflick limit: only one or two modifications can be made to the cells before they die out. For most tissues, moreover, there is as yet no reliable way to introduce the new cells so as to replace the faulty ones and make the desired correction.

The Hayflick limit is governed in the cell by repetitive DNA division counters, called *telomeres*, located at the ends of the chromosomes. During each cell division some of the telomeres break off. Below a certain threshold, the reduction in the number of telomeres activates genes that cause the cell to self-destruct. Researchers recently have learned how to produce an enzyme, telomerase, that resets this "death clock" by restoring the telomeres. In time, study of the enzyme may allow us to rejuvenate human cells at will and thus change a larger number of genes without running afoul of the Hayflick limit.

A great deal of work has been and is being done to bring therapeutic genes into the body directly, either as naked DNA in solution to be absorbed through cell membranes, or by using various vectors. So far, most of them have not worked very well.

Yet there have been a few remarkable successes, such as the spectacular results that Dr. Alain Fischer and his colleagues at Paris's Hospital Necker reported in April 2000. They cured two infants of severe combined immunodeficiency (SCID).

This syndrome results from the immune system's total failure to develop, caused by a defective gene on the X chromosome. It quickly ends in death from the slightest infection unless the child is kept in a completely sterile environment—a sterile bubble, hence the term "bubble babies." In normal development, progenitor cells in the bone marrow give rise to all of the various white blood cells of a healthy immune system. The key to treatment is the fact that progenitor cells with the proper gene naturally and aggressively replace the defective cells without further intervention if they are merely placed in the baby's bloodstream. In this case, doctors used a vector, a retrovirus, to bring the therapeutic genes into some of the babies' defective progenitor cells in vitro, then cultured and injected them.

The Stem-Cell Dilemma

Unfortunately, most diseases are not so accommodating. Spurred by several recent achievements, however, biologists seem likely quite soon to solve many of the problems of delivering therapeutic genes. Methods developed in 1999 for culturing human embryonic stem cells will eventually combine with emergent technologies for controlling their differentiation into specific kinds of tissue; this will allow biologists to make the raw material for repairs throughout the body. Right now, however, scientists are still grappling with challenges arising from the complexity of the stem-cell growth process.

Embryonic stem cells stand at the beginning of the developmental process, changing in response to genetically programmed chemical signals to become all the cell types in the body as the fetus develops. Thousands of research groups are studying the chemicals that control these changes. Japanese scientists recently showed they could prod frog embryonic cells to grow complete eyes or ears merely by exposing them to two different concentrations of retinoic acid, a compound that the body makes from vitamin A. Another group has stimulated mouse embryonic stem cells to form the myelin-producing sheath cells that surround nerve fibers, a discovery offering potential hope to sufferers of multiple sclerosis, in which the myelin sheaths are destroyed.

Others have found a "gatekeeper protein" called Oct-3/4, which at different concentrations tells embryonic stem cells whether to make placenta, differentiated body cells, or more stem cells. A group at Ohio State University is one of several working on developing a *bioreactor*, a support medium or tissue matrix for growing stem cells outside the body and organizing them into simple artificial tissue. Using spongy, nutrient-soaked polyester as a support medium, they found that they could modify intercellular signaling, and thus differentiation, by "squeezing the sponge"–varying the pressure to vary the distance between cells. Eventually such techniques will let technicians grow supplies of any cell type, even those that do not normally divide after differentiation, such as heart muscle and neurons.

Scientists eager to study embryonic stem cells have encountered much opposition. Since the embryo is destroyed in the process of harvesting stem cells from it, many people believe that such research might increase the abortion rate or create "conception mills" that would buy donated eggs and sperm to make embryos for resale to laboratories. In August 2001, President George

W. Bush okayed federal funding of research using preexisting stem cell lines–renewable stocks of embryonic cells that had already been harvested. The decision established a firm legal foundation for a minimum level of basic research on embryonic stem cells. As of this writing, the terrorist attacks of September 11, 2001, have led to an indefinite postponement of debate on expanded research involving creation of new cell lines.

However, discovery of stem cells in adults may be invalidating objections to such research anyway. The human body seems tremendously eager to help. Researchers have found stem cells hidden in bone marrow, skin, muscle, even in tissues previously thought to have no regenerative capacity whatsoever, such as the retina of the eye, and the brain. Implants of neural stem cells have partially regrown severed spinal cords in rats. Stem cells have been isolated from the placenta and from fat, raising the possibility that both normal birth and liposuction could be commercial sources of stem cells.

But there are stem cells and there are stem cells–at least in the normal development of the body. *Totipotent* stem cells are the fertilized egg and its first few daughter cells, which together are called the blastocyst. This small blob of totipotent cells gives rise to the placenta, all the cells of the adult body, and more stem cells, pluripotent and multipotent cells. *Pluripotent* stem cells are from the inner cell mass of the blastocyst stage; they become the adult body; they no longer form cells of the placenta, which develops from the blastocyst's outer envelope cells.

Multipotent stem cells are partially differentiated, tissue-specific cells that have traveled partway down the path of differentiation toward one of the two hundred specialized human cell types. As the fetus and then the infant grows, they develop further into the fully developed cells of each organ system–bone, muscle, blood, and so on. Some of them are held in reserve in adult tissues.

Until recently, this journey toward differentiation was thought to be irreversible. One of the biggest surprises to come from the latest research is that this gradation of stem-cell potency may be an illusion. It turns out that tissue-specific stem cells can do more than replenish adult cells within their own clan. Several laboratories have shown that, given the right growth factors, stem cells from one part of the body can fully regress to the embryonic stage, then develop into completely different stem and tissue cells. This discovery may render moot the objections of fetal-rights advocates against research using human embryonic stem cells.

Given the proper stimulus in the lab, muscle stem cells, at least in mice, form platelets, red corpuscles, and the full array of white blood cells, all of which are normally generated only in bone marrow or spleen.

Also in mice, blood stem cells from bone marrow have been transplanted into the liver, where they turned into fully functional liver cells and corrected experimentally induced liver failure. Since blood travels throughout the body, some biologists think it includes a chemical system that senses which organs need a supply of new cells and then triggers stem cells to produce replacements. If so, corrective genes one day may be inserted into stem cells and delivered naturally to their target tissue by the blood, making the hazardous and complicated use of altered viruses or other vectors unnecessary for genetic therapy.

Another major obstacle to genetic therapy is the difficulty of populating the target tissue with new cells without having to kill off the old ones in a dangerous way. Doctors today transplant bone marrow only after destroying the dysfunctional blood-producing cells in the patient's own marrow. Sometimes the result— in leukemia, sickle-cell anemia, and other blood diseases—is spectacular, but 10 percent of the patients die, and those who live are often severely debilitated for a long time, first by the marrow- killing chemicals or radiation and then by transplant-rejection crises and the required immune-suppressant drugs. Only in last- ditch therapies can such risks be tolerable.

Another crucial area of ignorance stands between us and our visions of an omnipotent medicine: the "command and control" system that organizes cells into tissues. Tissue engineers must not only mix the correct types of cells in the correct numbers but also must provide the proper cues to cause them to divide at the cor- rect rate for the correct number of times; then other cues to cause them to link with other cells and form the correct three-di- mensional architecture; while at the same time infiltrating the new tissue with blood vessels, lymph channels, and nerve fibers. Learning to speak the language, chemical and possibly electrical, by which the body does this job during its growth phase remains a task at least as formidable as mapping the human genome.

One more new technology may be crucial to integrating vari- ous strains of knowledge into a universally effective genetic med- icine. Investigators at several labs are working on methods to transfer a complete nucleus from one cell to another. Under proper conditions, the cell body reprograms the nuclear genome so that the two work together as though they were made for each other in the first place. In time, geneticists may be able to take nuclei containing a genetic correction from differentiated cells of the desired tissue type and insert them into stem cells from the patient's own body, guaranteeing that the new tissue grown from them will be immunologically compatible and not rejected.

Bright Skies Ahead?

Despite gaps in our knowledge, many therapies based on genetics will be available very soon. Largely as a result of mapping the human genome, physicians now see clear research paths toward vastly improved treatments and eventual cures for nearly every disease known.

Here is a sampling of some of the medical breakthroughs we can expect in the first two decades of the new millennium:

- Genome maps of hundreds of disease bacteria—including those that cause syphilis, gonorrhea, cholera, and meningitis—are giving chemists leads for new antibiotics that will be more effective without causing side effects. Even a cure for malaria, the world's leading killer, is in the cards. An entirely new type of antibiotic derived from protegrins, proteins found in white blood cells, promises to be effective against viral diseases, as traditional antibiotics are not.
- Vaccines against numerous diseases, even tooth decay and the common cold, are being developed.
- New antidepressants may help the approximately 40 percent of patients for whom current drugs fail. New painkillers affecting the intracellular messenger system promise more relief with fewer side effects.
- New tests for drug-detoxification enzymes in the liver should help eliminate most of the estimated 100,000 to 300,000 deaths that occur each year in the United States from adverse reactions to medicines, and even some of the 10,000 deaths from overdoses of illegal drugs.

- New "designer estrogens" will be better at preventing postmenopausal hot flashes, vaginal dryness, mood swings, osteoporosis, and heart attacks—without raising the risk of blood clots and breast or uterine cancer, as current estrogen-replacement drugs do.
- A cure for type I (juvenile-onset) diabetes using transplants of laboratory-grown insulin-producing cells seems likely to be one of the first fruits of research on embryonic stem cells.
- Several types of drugs are being developed to treat parkinsonism and Alzheimer's disease. Other researchers are seeking cures via lab-grown neurons transplanted into the brain. Further in the future, nerve growth factors may be used to augment the size and connectivity of specific neuron groups anywhere in the brain.
- Scientists are closing in on a vaccine against AIDS and a cure for the early stages of the disease.
- Microelectronic devices and implants of living cells will give near-perfect sight to the blind and hearing to the deaf.
- Microelectronics and nerve growth factors will completely repair the spinal damage that causes paraplegia.
- Tissue engineering, the art of creating artificial flesh and organs from combinations of synthetic materials and living cells, will make transplants of various body parts common-place. Artificial skin is already revolutionizing the treatment of severe burns. Next on the list are cartilage to repair arthritis damage, then teeth, breasts, and livers, and eventually hearts and lungs, and even parts of the brain.
- An array of the body's own cell growth factors, artificially produced, will heal wounds and debilitating injuries as good as new, without scars.

- Growth factors and gene injections have already been used in a prototype treatment to produce new coronary arteries, as mentioned above. Drugs to remove deposits of arterio-sclerotic plaque, as well as transplants of lab-grown cardiac tissue, and eventually entire hearts, promise a repertoire of effective treatments for heart disease.
- Study of the human genome shows that about one fifth of all our genes code for hormones and other signaling molecules. Many of these are overproduced in various cancers. Hundreds of new cancer drugs will emerge from work on these genes in the next 10 years.
- Cures are also in the works for emphysema, rheumatoid arthritis, lupus erythematosis, psoriasis, osteoporosis, and many other diseases.

In the moderately distant future—let's guess 20 to 50 years—a person's entire genome might be routinely upgraded or rejuvenated by means of stem cells. Individual genes would be knocked out and replaced to repair or improve certain tissues; the new replacement cells would be cultured in the lab, then seeded back into the client. Such methods promise indefinite prolongation of life without aging. In time, "genetic cassettes" of customized chromosomes promise a virtually unlimited array of somatic upgrades.

In terms of science, then, the forecast for medicine looks bright and sunny. In terms of delivering the miracles fairly and efficiently to the people who need them, however, the forecast is rain, possibly heavy at times. It is to this severe weather that we wish to draw your attention in the rest of our book.

Too Much
of a Good Thing

UNFORTUNATELY, THE AWESOME POWERS of the new medicine are being entrusted to a dysfunctional system. Though rich in technology, American health care too often leaves both patient and doctor ill served. By all statistical measures, notably infant mortality and adult life expectancy, the American system of health care is worse at maintaining public health than is medicine in most other industrialized nations. On the personal level, it's too cumbersome. It costs way too much, and even so it doesn't come close to serving everyone who needs care.

There are many reasons that modern American medicine costs more and satisfies less. Fraud and inflated malpractice settlements are often blamed, but actually they are not major causes. On the basis of federal statistics and assuming slow economic growth in 2001, we estimate for 2002, in 2002 dollars, a health-care bill of $1.9 trillion, or 18 percent of our gross domestic product (GDP), which is projected to be $10.5 trillion. Litigation related to medical practice eats up about $40 billion a year. Fraud by both patients and providers, though harder to estimate, probably adds $100 billion or so. Together, these two factors account for a little more than 7 percent of health-care outlays. They flourish in the already overheated climate of American medicine's commercialized confusion. Other nations spend much less per capita for health care yet have fewer rip-offs and lawsuits.

Administrative expenses, conservatively estimated at $250 billion dollars, account for a larger share of the burden, about 14 percent. So by cutting administrative costs in half, we'd save another 7 percent or so.

Nevertheless, the chief problem is the American approach to medicine per se. Our medicine is top-heavy. We buy too many expensive machines and drugs, and we train too many specialists, an astounding three fourths of all our doctors. Owing to our structure of financial rewards, we have too few general practitioners, especially outside the cities, and an ever-dwindling supply of *experienced* GPs able to pass along to the younger generation a lifetime's accumulated wisdom about what really works in day-to-day treatment of the most typical ailments.

With so much specialized medical personnel and machinery available, it's probably inevitable that it is used even when it's not appropriate. As a result, roughly half of the most expensive treatments in the United States are unnecessary, even by medicine's own criteria. This figure is no idle guess. Between 1984 and 1994, a landmark series of investigations, led by Dr. Robert Brook for the Rand Corporation, focused on some of the most common surgical procedures, including angioplasty, coronary bypass, hysterectomy, and gallbladder removal. Analyzing their results conservatively, Brook and his colleagues concluded that one fourth to one third of the procedures were either totally unjustified or entailed risks that equaled or outweighed any potential benefit. The raw numbers suggested that the unneeded operations were more like half of the total.

Other studies support the same conclusion. In 1991, for example, a major analysis by Millimann & Roberts, a large firm of accountants and benefits consultants, found that 53 percent of both inpatient and outpatient care in the United States was "medically unnecessary."

This gross overmedication results from a synergistic mix of factors. It involves unavoidable givens of American history and culture, combined with the universals of human psychology, all intertwined with legislative mistakes and—perhaps most important of all—the power of money.

The Best-Laid Plans

Insurance and medicine first became partners in the United States during the 1930s. Before then, most middle-class families could absorb the costs of at least a short hospital stay without facing the specter of bankruptcy. Then the Great Depression left millions of Americans unable to pay any medical bills at all. By 1933, over 400 hospitals had gone under.

Communities searching for a solution for this economic and social calamity thought they saw one in the Baylor University Hospital Plan, which had been developed in 1929 by Justin Ford Kimball, formerly superintendent of the Dallas public school system and then vice president of Baylor University. His idea, the first modern health-insurance scheme, was to cover all local teachers with medical insurance for hospitalization. Soon other groups of employees were added, and the idea of prepaid premiums for entry to a shared-risk pool spread quickly to other communities. The Baylor plan became the prototype for Blue Cross and all similar arrangements for hospital insurance. Endorsement by the American Medical Association in 1938 made it a national standard and led most insurance companies to offer competing policies.

Wage controls put in place during World War II meant that medical benefits were left as the main bargaining point between unions and management. In response, a few labor unions and companies began devising systems to cover all medical expenses, not just hospitalization. In general, these early plans were straightforward contracts that bought discounted medical services by the year and provided them to members for a flat rate, which stayed the same whether or not one needed a doctor in any given year. Such arrangements worked because they saved money for both labor and management, and they weren't designed to generate profits for anyone. There were no hidden costs, no complicated limits on coverage, no executive bonuses tied to company stock prices, and little room for fraud.

The most successful of these nonprofit health plans was California's Kaiser Permanente, begun for Henry Kaiser's shipyard and mill workers in the San Francisco Bay area. The Kaiser plan was the first, and for a long time one of the few, to cover all medical care. In addition, Kaiser Permanente acquired its own medical facilities, thus becoming, in effect, the first health maintenance organization, although that term wasn't coined for another 30 years. It streamlined the setup further by emphasizing primary care over specialization, thus promoting health and reducing the fee-for-service dynamic in which doctors prosper most by doing the costliest procedures.

Today, Kaiser Permanente remains the largest, and by most measures the best, of the few HMOs that still follow the nonprofit model. Much of the following discussion does not apply to them.

In these early years, insurance payments were based on hospitals' standard rates, determined by demand on a break-even basis. The risks were spread evenly among the pool of customers in each region, a practice known as community rating. Doctors' fees, usually not covered by insurance, were limited by what people could afford.

Soon after the war, laws exempting nonprofit health plans from state insurance premium taxes further encouraged the growth of Blue Cross and Blue Shield. With more volume to offer, the Blues bargained for hospital discount rates, and in return were able to accept all who applied, without limits on age or current health status. Soon the majority of consumers had hospital coverage of some kind.

The idea of risk-sharing among subscribers to a commercial (for-profit) or semicommercial (controlled-profit) medical insurance plan caught on fast. However, the idea of mandating some sort of universal health-care coverage encountered much more resistance. During the Depression, and even during the wartime and postwar prosperity, there had always been a substantial minority who could not afford hospital insurance or more than very low doctor bills. Nonetheless, the AMA opposed all attempts to lower doctor and hospital costs or legislate coverage. The doctors' association turned down a 1932 plan to promote group practice and resource-sharing among its members, even calling supporters "medical soviets."

In late 1945, President Truman proposed a plan for national health insurance that would have covered a short list of basic medical services for all citizens. This decentralized plan, which would have allowed consumers free choice of doctors, called for a 4 percent health tax on the first $3,600 of income. The AMA's reaction to this initiative was to hire the California public relations firm of Whitaker & Baxter to mount a national ad campaign based on the theme that national health insurance was the first domino falling toward totalitarian communism. Led by the AMA's spokesman, Morris Fishbein, whose column ran in almost every daily paper in the land for a quarter century, the campaign scuttled Truman's initiative with a withering barrage of propaganda against "socialized medicine." What physicians feared most in Truman's initiative was that some of their fees would be controlled.

For the next two decades, the American medical system remained one of direct economic stratification ("You get what you can pay for"), run by a guild of independent entrepreneurs in uneasy alliance with the growing empire of private insurance companies.

Something eventually had to be done to help the elderly and the poor, who often could not afford the new wonder drugs and surgeries emerging from the postwar research labs. In 1965 Medicare and Medicaid changed the game.

Unfortunately, in creating these new government programs, "mistakes were made," as the saying goes. To overcome the physicians' fear of socialized medicine (i.e., control of fees), Congress set reimbursement at "usual and customary" rates, giving providers the collective ability to charge whatever they wanted; ironically, the new programs meant that they were largely freed from the normal competitive constraints of a free-market system. Likewise, hospitals were allowed to fold capital expansion costs into their rates, giving them an incentive to grow regardless of need. Furthermore, Congress soon allocated money to double the annual number of medical school graduates, who created new services to keep themselves busy in a nation where consumers were eager to buy and taxpayers were forced to foot the bill.

In 1968, spending on medical care consumed 6.3 percent of America's gross domestic product. This seemed exorbitant at the time, and as a result we began our experiment in what came to be called "managed care." This is a collective term for various systems of institutional channels and barriers between health-care providers and their patients. The first and most common of these systems are the aforementioned health maintenance organizations (HMOs), although there are others. In 1973 Congress passed the Health Maintenance Organization Act, enabling legislation that established a program of grants and loans for HMO start-ups. The law also specified minimum levels of medical benefits that must be offered by HMOs bidding on government contracts. The basic design was a closed system, an "all under one roof" health-care complex or a chain of linked facilities that offered members a complete menu of health-care services in return for a monthly fee and, usually, a specified co-payment for each service. It was modeled on the Kaiser Permanente plan and a few others, notably the clinic system in Palo Alto, California.

There was one crucial new twist in the legislation, however: HMOs could choose to do business as investor-owned, for-profit companies.

Turn the Kaiser-style union-company plan into a moneymaking enterprise and you have the modern corporate HMO. During the eighties, the further evolution of the corporate HMO proceeded largely according to the "managed competition" model of Alain Enthoven, a Stanford University economics professor and former Pentagon systems analyst who had helped Robert McNamara decide which weapons to buy for use against Vietnam.

The idea of managed competition is to combine "market forces"–the profit imperative and the tight cost controls presumably common in business–with cooperation among all HMOs in a city or region when it came to purchasing equipment and services, so as to get volume discounts. In theory this would give the aggregated HMOs monopolistic buying power while leaving enough competition between individual plans to induce them to squeeze out nonessential procedures (and patients), thereby reducing total costs, even once a slice of profit for the investors had been factored in. Though not thoroughly applied by government mandate, the system has been approximated in some areas by corporate mergers and alliances.

Managed competition eventually became the core of Hillary Clinton's health-care reform proposal, during the first Clinton administration.

The Maslow Memorial Medical Theme Park

These policy errors–the AMA's resistance to a national health plan, the creation of Medicare and Medicaid with built-in cost-inflation incentives, and the linkage of the HMO idea with for-profit corporations–exacerbated the overgrowth of medicine in the latter half of the twentieth century. They did not, however, cause it. Predisposing cultural factors had existed for centuries.

Modern medical practice has its roots in a series of cultural, social, and economic changes that profoundly shaped Western civilization over a period of four hundred years. During the Renaissance, widespread persecution of midwives and herbalists as witches had almost entirely eliminated traditional village healers, most of whom were women, in the countries of Western Europe. Their function had been to foster the health of whole persons in close-knit communities, using knowledge of plant remedies accumulated since prehistoric times and more or less available to all at minimal cost.

Then, from the late seventeenth century through the nineteenth century, the Industrial Revolution destroyed the traditional sense of community that had held together the agricultural and feudal societies of medieval and Renaissance Europe. With the spread of modern capitalism, workers became largely anonymous, interchangeable units of labor. As a result, traditional forms of family life were greatly weakened as well. The social changes almost completely removed fathers from the home except while they were sleeping. Parents and children were separated from each other in distant factories. The fact that children later were remanded from factory to school did not change the basic situation. The young could no longer be with their elders and watch them at work. The cost in mental health has been incalculable.

Modern medicine conformed to the new social order. Using techniques and assumptions drawn from experimental science, it dealt with isolated organs–parts of people, who themselves came to be considered parts of giant commercial machines. It aimed to fix time-pressed workers' symptoms so as to get them back into production quickly. To do so, it relied more and more on concentrated extracts or chemically synthesized drugs rather than herbs in their natural state—for example, digitalis instead of foxglove, from which it comes. These new drugs were available only from professionals at high prices.

Fast-forward to the late twentieth and early twenty-first centuries. Both industry and industrialized medicine have grown so big we find it hard to imagine any other system. In the developed nations, a bourgeois majority concentrates on ascending the stations of wage servitude from entry-level hell to the paradise of wealth. To survive this "rat race," we seem to need a lot of medicine to keep us functioning and conventionally sane. Plus, adequate health care has become one of the major rewards of success.

In his 1962 classic, *Toward a Psychology of Being*, Abraham Maslow proposed a broader view of human aspiration. He broke away from the illness-oriented psychology of his day, which assumed that the troubled client was crazy and needed to "adjust" to society. Instead, Maslow constructed a theory of mental *health* and ways of attaining it. He postulated a hierarchy of needs motivating all activity. These needs are usually diagrammed as a five-level pyramid, beginning with physiological requirements (food, water, health) at the base and progressing through safety (shelter, protection, community) to love (friendship, sexuality, romance, family) and esteem (the respect of peers), culminating in self-actualization (creative work and subjective fulfillment).

Like all schemata, Maslow's hierarchy is simpler than life. It suggests that some needs are "lower" and that these *must* be satisfied before the "higher" rewards are available. In reality, people tend to get what they can wherever they can find it, even under the most adverse conditions of poverty and oppression.

Still, Maslow's pyramid gives an intuitive clarity to the goals we all try to meet. It's much like the *gradus ad Parnassum*, the journey up Parnassus (the Greek mountain sacred to the Muses) to a fully realized artistic life, which symbolized similar goals for Renaissance people.

Along with Carl Rogers, Rollo May, and others, Maslow founded a humanistic psychology, one that saw life as an unfolding or flowering, driven initially by normal bodily desires and fueled at the upper levels by psychic energy derived from peak experiences—all the forms of religious, athletic, sexual, artistic, social, pharmacologic, or meditative at-one-ment or "flow." Maslow emphasized the role of curiosity and the sense of beauty in motivating people to achieve.

It was like Freud in color. Founded upon the primacy of the individual and the assumption of free will, Maslow's ideas, much filtered and elaborated, have been so widely disseminated among educators, marketers, social and political leaders, and the health-care establishment as to become our mythology, the foremost belief system of the consumer state. Most Americans and Western Europeans now take it as an article of faith not only that the ultimate goal of life is self-fulfillment but that this goal is achievable.

Maslow's is an optimistic, open-hearted philosophy. However, as popularized, it also tends to suggest that humans consist of an unlimited number of economic receptor sites at which the five levels of need can be redirected into the desire for merchandise. And in a capitalist society, it's probably inevitable that this slant on Maslow should predominate.

The economist's word for desire is "demand," and the ideal of self-fulfillment creates a very demanding society, especially given the aging of the population and the lengthening of productive life past maturity. We have more time to want more. For perhaps the first time in history, most of the population expects to "have it all" in a way that used to be possible only for social and economic elites. It's no coincidence that per capita consumption of goods and services in the United States has doubled since 1957.

This evolution in social and economic expectations was bound to have an impact on health care. In the past, Western medicine concerned itself with the physiological level and, to a lesser extent, with safety needs by way of advances in public health, epidemiology, and disease prevention. Now, medicine's aspirations are rapidly climbing Maslow's pyramid. Viagra follows birth control and breast reconfiguration as a medical aid toward fulfillment of love needs. Psychiatric drugs and psychotherapy are medicine's still-primitive tools for helping people find self-esteem and self-actualization.

In the future, the emphasis of medicine will shift toward more and better ways to promote satisfaction of the upper-level needs. Genetic and biochemical research will enable this shift; the profit motive will drive it. Naturally the health-care industry will concentrate on those with the most money to spend.

Molecular medicine hopes to be, and probably will be, the culmination of the trend advanced by Viagra—a desire for every drug and a drug for every desire. Mix in the high-stakes competition for profits reminiscent of a frontier-style gold rush, plaster the virtual fences with ads to beef up demand, and you have the modern medical carnival: a theme park where every barker promises the ride of a lifetime.

The Generation of Medicine

The medical sector of the American economy also is being expanded by a demographic bulge. The Baby Boom generation, those born between 1946 and 1963, moves through the health-care system like a pig in a python, consuming a disproportionate share of resources because of its disproportionate size compared with other generations older and younger. But instead of becoming smaller as it's digested, this metaphoric pig expands as it gets older and requires more medical care.

The Census Bureau and the Social Security Administration predict a dramatic rise in the proportion of our population over age 65 during the next three or four decades. Federal planners expect average life spans to lengthen into the eighties, and a recent private study suggests that their forecasts are too conservative by 5 to 10 percent, even without taking account of future advances in longevity medicine.

Increased longevity already is bringing to some an expanded freedom to play a variety of roles in the course of a life. It no longer seems quite so unusual for people to enter law school or set themselves up as self-employed business owners in their fifties, after raising a family or putting in a full term of corporate service.

One of the biggest changes of the next few decades will be the shift away from retirement toward a new career in later life. Far from being a burden, older workers are becoming a national resource, but it will be one of public policy's greatest challenges to make gainful employment available for them and meet their ongoing medical needs.

Although an increasing number of people will elect to work past the age of 65, by 2050 nonworking retirees may outnumber workers in some countries, notably the United States and Japan, with dire long-term consequences for both public and private pension plans as well as the health-care system. Although many financially secure older people will be enjoying their longer lives in unprecedented good health, a large percentage, living in poverty and/or isolation, will not, and so a larger portion of our population than ever will consist of disabled elderly persons needing constant medical care. The Department of Health and Human Services expects demand for nursing homes, for example, to double or triple by 2030.

Besides being the largest American generation ever, the Baby Boomers are, as a group, the most privileged ever. They grew up in the early postwar empire when the United States was undisputed king of the world. Their formative years, the 1950s and early 1960s, were an era now often called the Golden Age of Medicine, when new drugs and surgeries gave physicians powers they'd never had before, exercised in an environment where the costs of health care hadn't yet become a major economic issue.

As the Boomers came of age during the economic expansion and transcendental idealism of the sixties, they enjoyed unprecedented sexual freedom, thanks in large measure to the birth control pill. Compared with the remembered past, medicine then seemed omnipotent, and it was still affordable. No wonder the Boomers grew up believing that, for them, the world was essentially without limits. So now, when something goes wrong in their (our) bodies, they (we) expect the repair team right away— and without undue fiscal sacrifice. To this extent, today's medicine is suffering from its own success.

In the seventies (which in social and psychological terms were actually a continuation of the sixties), the human-potential movement put the finishing touches on Baby Boomers' entitlement syndrome. Maslow's humanistic psychology—popularized—became the grail of human perfectibility.

Philosophically, this is an ideal. Psychologically, it's a macro—an automated routine that does a complex task at the push of a button. When applied to economics, it creates (among other results) an exponentially growing appetite for health care. If happiness hasn't come from material success, then mental or physical self-improvement may provide it. Better yet, that process can be brought under medicine's aegis—literally, its shield—to protect the customer in what otherwise would be a lonelier, more uncertain quest. Physical and mental problems and limitations that in other cultures would be accepted without question as simply "part of life" are in this environment seen as fixable—an outlook that may seem heroic or misguided, depending on your bias, but one that is unquestionably expensive.

In the eighties, the nation embraced a purely materialistic view of the Maslovian goals. Business bought whole sectors of society not previously for sale, notably much of the penal and medical systems. It redoubled its successful efforts, begun in earnest about 1950, to channel all of the human desires symbolized by the Maslow pyramid through the sluice of advertising into demand for specific goods and services. Central to the entire project is the implied corollary that there is nothing *outside* the universe of product, no goal or desire that cannot be fulfilled through a purchase.

Finally, the nineties were like the eighties with a better actor in the lead. The short-lived health-care reform show that the Clinton years began with achieved precisely nothing, while medicine as business enjoyed tremendous prosperity. The natural-foods and self-health movements and the tiny minority of people who seek a frugal life close to the earth have been the only (negligible) restraint on the expansion of medical costs.

We're generalizing, of course, which is always risky. But it seems fair to say that the United States in the early years of the twenty-first century is a land in which most people want and expect to use every new tool available to ease their suffering and improve their lives. Developers of the new tools want to sell as many of them as possible. The doctor often owns stock in one of the tool companies and steers patients toward needless, expensive purchases that fill his or her pockets twice, a process called self-referral. Thus do cultural and economic forces reinforce each other, making the lust for medicine grow faster than the population.

Now, just after the turn of the millennium, the cost of our health-care system has reached 18 percent of GDP. A recent report written by Sheila Smith for the Department of Health and Human Services predicts that our total medical bill will double in the next decade, passing $2.1 trillion in 2007. Smith's report assumes that continued economic expansion will keep medicine's share of the economy at 18 percent, but a recession could dramatically increase that figure, since demand for health care tends to rise regardless of economic fluctuations.

Thus, medicine has become the economic equivalent of the expanding universe. It consumes a larger share of our society's wealth and energy than did pyramid building in ancient Egypt or the construction of cathedrals in medieval Europe. Some financial prophets see medicine constituting one fourth or even one third of our economy in the second decade of the current century.

The Medical Fix

Medicalization–the proliferation of services offered by physicians–may be the most important cause of increased health-care costs.

Medicalization works in several ways. One aspect of it is the phenomenon of specialists subdividing the available fields into ever-smaller parcels. For example, adolescent medicine developed as a separate specialty only when pediatricians began running out of younger patients, in the 1980s. Similarly, cardiology is now split into invasive and noninvasive branches. Of course, it's natural that the more narrowly specialties are defined, the more problems are discovered within each specialty and the more specialized treatments are demanded to solve those problems.

Medicalization also happens when physicians claim more aspects of human life as their turf, turning commonplace conditions into "diseases" that can be cured only by medicine. Menstruation, routine childbirth, everyday aches and pains, sexual behavior both "normal" and "abnormal," gambling, substance abuse, aging, and other physical and emotional problems we used to tackle with the help of friends, families, and lovers all have become the doctor's business. This is not to say that medicine may not be able to help. The question is, how much help can we afford?

Death has become almost infinitely medicalized. Hospitals routinely spend a quarter of their budgets on critical care, most of which goes to elderly patients in the last few days of life. As a nation, we spend $20 billion to $30 billion a year operating life-support systems for people in coma, most of whom never wake up. The practice of "churning" the dying with tests and treatments to run up billings, over protests by patient and family, is an underreported national scandal.

Naturally this is one of the most emotional issues health-care practitioners face. Friends and lovers of the dying often are unwilling to give up hope. Medicine's readiness to try any measure to save the patient, expense be damned, always has been one of its noblest and most cherished ideals. Today, however, now that measures and expenses both have grown to unforeseen proportions, more and more people agree that heroic efforts to stave off death, especially when the patient is moribund at an advanced age–even begging for release–should not be routine.

Medicine also expands by a sort of technological tumescence. Research constantly gives doctors new methods, new things to try. Often only experience can decide whether a novel technology is useful (to say nothing of cost-effective) in pursuing the presumed goal of health. However, now that medicine is more a business than a service, it increasingly accepts the logic of capitalism, which requires growth at all costs. Merely sustaining a market or, worse, shrinking it, is never acceptable to investors. For them, a sudden outbreak of health would be disastrous.

Yet over and over again we let ourselves believe the promise that we'll "save money through technology." This myth is to medicine what the "paperless office" is to computerized business. Both fables ignore the fact that technology has a life of its own, creating new expectations to fill new capacities.

The predicted savings never materialize because in a private system every hospital or medical practice must compete with every other hospital or practice in a region. Thus, instead of Eastside Hospital buying the $10 million NMR imager and Westside getting the new PET scanner (and dividing the patient population amicably between them), both hospitals have to buy both machines (and compete for patients). Rather than economies of scale, we have the math of aggregation, in which the total cost reflects not actual demand but rather the sum of the fantasies all the competitors have of dominating the market.

Now add the paradigm of permanent progress. New machinery seldom lives out its full service life. The pace of technological change and the pressure of competition dictate that both Eastside and Westside must replace their equipment with the latest models before they've realized the profits that otherwise would have come after paying the old machines off. But those profits can't be sacrificed; they must now come from higher charges to patients. Likewise, the price of a drug must reflect not only the expense of research and clinical testing; it must also take into account an ever shorter market life between years of trials and the next hot molecule down the pipeline.

Here's an example: Since the first experimental transplant of a chimpanzee kidney into a human by Dr. Keith Reemtsma in 1963, an enormous amount of research has gone into using pigs as a source of organs for humans. Now, work on using embryonic stem cells to grow new organs may make xenotransplantation obsolete just as the field is about to reach success. The knowledge gained may have other uses, but still, all that effort and money, in terms of what society might have done with it, will have been wasted. Without a coherent plan for cultivating technology to meet social rather than financial needs, we'll be throwing away half the money we spend on our new medicine, just as we do on the old.

Take Two Options and
Don't Call Me in the Morning

Any study of medical economics is bound to lead to a certain fatalism. As a result of the factors we've just described, and despite all attempts to rein it in during the last three decades, medicine's share of gross domestic product has risen inexorably by one percentage point every five years.

This process did not go unnoticed in the financial markets, and during the eighties investors quietly bought one third of our health-care system from communities and nonprofit boards and turned the institutions into profit centers. The process continues apace, and today medicine has been almost entirely transformed from a service industry into an investment vehicle. Margin has triumphed over mission with little public discussion of what that change has meant.

To paraphrase Calvin Coolidge, the business of medicine is now business. Most doctors and nurses remain as dedicated as ever, but we sense the cold eyes of the speculator looking over their shoulders. We long for bygone warmth, but we might as well ask our stockbroker to make house calls.

Egregious stonewalling and denial of care in order to cut costs have been well publicized as tactics used by some HMOs. One can argue that the search for bottom-line efficiency leads inevitably to suboptimal care across the board. Certainly there are some disturbing statistics to support that view. For-profit HMOs spend 6.3 percent less of their total revenue on "medical losses"—in other words, treatment—than do the nonprofits. From 1983 to 1993, during the first wave of transition to an investor-owned medical system, the number of Americans who died each year from medication errors jumped 260 percent.

Yet so far, in the day-to-day world of patient care, most for-profit providers seem to work much the same as the nonprofits do. Nonprofits even generate the same level of "surplus" in many cases. The critical difference is that for them the returns are optional and are used for research or to subsidize low-cost care to the poor, whereas for-profits *must* satisfy investors, owners, managers, and financial agents from their revenues. The history of the Hospital Corporation of America (HCA), one of the first for-profit hospital chains, illustrates the point perfectly.

HCA's Chairman, Dr. Thomas Frist, Jr., and several colleagues started the company in 1986 with one hospital in Nashville. By February 1992, when the company went public, it was managing several hundred hospitals with annual revenues of over $5 billion.

Much of the company's profit making happened in 1989, when HCA's management dumped their poorly performing hospitals and negotiated a leveraged buyout of $5.1 billion against future revenues, arranging a rich payday for founders, shareholders, and the investment firms that handled the transaction. Among the latter, Goldman Sachs received 10 million shares of stock and $7.75 million cash for helping to manage and underwrite the deal. For handling the issue of private stock as part of the buyout, HCA paid Morgan Guaranty $50 million. Frist himself bought $33 million in shares at that time, which were worth $280 million three years later. Cashing in $127 million of the bonanza made him the highest-paid executive in the United States that year.

How did all this prosperity affect medical care? It didn't benefit HCA's patients. They had already paid their money, recovered (or not), and left the hospitals, having received about the same level of care they would've gotten anywhere else.

It didn't benefit HCA's doctors and nurses. Most of them weren't investors, and they all continued to be paid about as much as their colleagues elsewhere.

Nor did this huge increase in value accrue to the communities in which HCA's hospitals are located, nor to the public at large. Most nonprofit facilities devote a substantial part of any surplus to research or low-cost programs for the poor. Most for-profits, like HCA, don't.

HCA's growth came from two main sources: stock appreciation and money from new investors. The increase in value of the stock derived from the corporation's success in maintaining a steadily increasing flow of revenue from patients. The new investment came mainly during the leveraged buyout, as management sold interests in the chain to speculators, who paid for their shares with other people's money borrowed from banks—just as executives of many companies did during the financial free-for-all of the Reagan years. Naturally the managers in such a transaction expect rewards for their sacrifice in selling the company on margin to outside forces. They generally receive a bonus, as well as stock options making them part owners.

In HCA's case, all of this gravy—options and incentives for managers, interest for bankers, fees for clever financial advisers, dividends and appreciation for shareholders, many of whom got their stock for free—all of it (except for leverage on the savings) came from the only source of revenue hospitals have: fees from patients. (Yes, there's interest income, but that comes from investing money from patients' fees.)

In other words, the $250 million made by Tom Frist, the millions made by his colleagues, Morgan Guaranty's $50 million, more millions for the bit players, and dividends for investors after the public offering—all of it came from extra payments made by patients over and above the actual cost of their treatment, either directly or (with an additional toll) through their insurers. Most galling of all, 40 percent of the profit enjoyed by this "private enterprise" came from taxes we all paid into Medicare and Medicaid.

Hillary Care: Opportunity Lost

The HMO idea was slow to catch on. Consumers worried that HMOs would provide lower-quality care than fee-for-service physicians, and businesspeople feared that setting up a complex medical-care and payment facility was too big a risk. As a result, during the mid- and late 1970s, Paul Ellwood, a physician and an originator of the HMO concept, invited prominent health-care policymakers to his home in Jackson Hole, Wyoming, several times a year for informal discussions about how to make the HMO concept more attractive.

This series of meetings came to focus primarily on how HMOs could succeed by making the practice of medicine more efficient. They could do this, several participants suggested, by means of "outcomes research"—statistical reviews of medical records to find out which treatments are cost-effective in a given situation and which are not. When such research considers outcomes over a long period of time, it can also help show which methods work well at maintaining subscribers' health and which are short-term fixes that cost more in the long run. At the urging of the Jackson Hole group, the Rand Corporation and other institutions conducted numerous large-scale studies of medical outcomes, the results of which have yet to be systematically applied to medical practice.

By the late 1980s, inexorable growth in medical costs had attracted much more interest from investors, and Dr. Ellwood convened a second series of meetings at his home. In keeping with the times, the conferees focused on financial and institutional strategies to save money.

Many gravitated to the Stanford economist Alain Enthoven's proposals for "managed competition," in which regional consortia of HMOs would compete with other such groups in a large area on the basis of the quality of their services and the discount prices they could offer as a result of their volume-buying power. Others thought that the idea amounted to little more than rearranging the deck chairs on the *Titanic*. However, Dr. Ellwood had invited executives from some of the major insurance companies to join the group, and they began to see how insurers could prosper by running HMOs if traditional insurance should become less rewarding.

Immediately after his inauguration in 1993, President Clinton set up his Task Force on National Health Care Reform. The group was led by a business consultant, Ira Magaziner, with Hillary Clinton serving as public spokesperson. It consisted of more than a hundred working members within the administration, who solicited input from several hundred additional experts.

The task force considered dozens of possibilities. Some of its members had become convinced that a centrally administered single-payer system like Canada's would be the best setup for a national health-care plan covering everyone. Indeed, such a law was proposed by Physicians for a National Health Program, based at Harvard, and was certified by the Congressional Budget Office as the simplest and most efficient of the seven or eight plans before the House.

In the end, though, the task force settled on an excruciatingly byzantine version of managed competition. The largest insurance companies would have had a tremendous advantage in setting up the huge regional HMO aggregates, called health insurance purchasing cooperatives (HIPCs) that the Clinton plan envisioned. These carriers—such as the Metropolitan Life, Aetna, Cigna, Travelers, and Prudential insurance companies—would make out just fine, whether the plan was adopted or rejected.

Thus the stage was set for rival ad campaigns. Hillary Clinton professed to champion the "little people" versus all insurance companies. The Health Insurance Association of America, which included the giants but also the medium-sized and small insurers who stood to lose out, weighed in with their "Harry and Louise" ads, which warned about loss of patients' right to choose their doctor. Predictably, neither side mentioned proposals to do away with the private insurance system altogether.

The complexity of managed competition helped turn the reform effort into an ideological battle. The proposed layers of giant companies owning smaller companies looked to those on the political left like a cave-in to business interests that would leave the public worse off than ever. The federal, state, and local agencies that were envisioned to oversee the HIPCs looked to the right like a web of bureaucracy that would also leave the public worse off than ever. Both sides were probably right.

In retrospect, the central failure of the whole process was the decision to keep the deliberations of the task force secret. This prevented informed public debate on the real issues and made a national consensus impossible. As a result, the decision by the House Ways and Means Committee to recommend none of the suggested plans for a vote by the House caused no great outcry.

During the last six months of 1993, medical industry contributions to the members of the House Ways and Means Committee amounted to $5.9 million, an average of $155,000 per member; 39 percent of these payments came from large insurance companies. Lawmakers tacitly agreed to pretend there was no alternative to the status quo but the President's plan, and Senator Bob Packwood wrote *finis* to the tale when he said, "We've killed healthcare reform. Now we've got to make sure our fingerprints aren't on it."

Thus passed the last consensus moment for a change. Consciously or not, Packwood also was speaking for the battalion of medical industry spin doctors who exploited public fears and prevented the real issues from entering the debate. These are the people President Carter had in mind back in the seventies when he said, "The health-care lobby is the most despicable on earth."

Reform thwarted, things stayed the same, only worse. Cost cutting (read: avoidance of service) by HMOs became a national disgrace. The resultant dip in their stock prices was an ironic outcome; the single-payer scare had led insurers to buy heavily into HMOs as sure-fire moneymakers. During the 1990s the conversion of all medical facilities to investor ownership neared completion; the results were predictable, and they were not pleasant.

The System We're Stuck With

Meanwhile, what happened to HCA? A new entity, Columbia/ HCA, was formed by the merger in 1994 of HCA with Columbia

Sunrise, a company begun in El Paso, Texas, in 1987 by a lawyer named Richard L. Scott. This company, in much the same way as HCA, was fruitful and multiplied. By 1997 the conglomerate comprised 342 hospitals (1 of every 20 in the country) and over 700 ancillary facilities, and its business had grown to $20 billion a year. That year, however, the pyramid began to crumble.

In the quest to continue the heady profit growth of the first few years, HCA's executives had turned to fraud, specifically systematic fraud of Medicare and other federal reimbursement programs on a scale never before uncovered.

HCA had spun off subsidiaries during the 1989 leveraged buyout, one of which was Quorum Health Group. Quorum brought its system of record keeping to (among many others) North Valley Hospital in Whitefish, Montana. There, a single honest accountant named James Alderson was fired for refusing to keep two sets of books. In late 1992, he filed a federal whistleblower suit under seal (i.e., a complaint made under various laws designed to protect employees from retaliation for exposing crimes by their employers), which flew below the radar through the Justice Department for five years before landing in the Columbia/HCA boardroom like a legal cruise missile. Scott and other executives golden-parachuted out.

In the ensuing trials, which are winding down as of this writing, several regional executives were convicted of fraud. Initial fines recovered approximately two thirds of the few million dollars those specific defendants had stolen. This return to the public treasury was, of course, reduced by the cost of investigating the crimes. Clyde Eder, the Quorum manager who'd fired Alderson, said in his deposition that the practice of keeping double books and defrauding the government was "common in the industry"—though now it may be less so for a while. (For the latest act in HCA's tawdry opera, as well as a more general consideration of the problem of medical fraud, please see Chapter 6.)

Today, as medical science begins to deliver its cabinetful of miracles, we remain cursed with a miracle-delivery system nobody likes except the few who own it. It is overpriced and inefficient, a rich mine for embezzlers and profiteers, an albatross we all carry around our bank accounts—and our lives.

Is this the system most of us want? The bottom-line question is whether medicine should be a business at all.

In contemporary America, this is a question that cannot be decided because it must not be asked. Our medicine *is* a business, and in the foreseeable future it will become ever more businesslike. Nevertheless, please keep the question in the back of your mind as you read the next few chapters, where we look at some of the other effects of medicine's continuing makeover.

CHAPTER 3

Gold in
Them Thar Ills

NOT ALL HEALTH-CARE EXPENSES show up on a balance sheet or in a cost-benefit analysis. Here we'll start to look at some of the hidden costs that result from commercializing medicine—losses both monetary and nonmonetary. Unregulated ruthless competition on the frontiers of science may conjure up romantic images of hardy men seeking their fortunes in Wild West gold rush days of yore, but in medicine the profiteering mentality has serious consequences—for medicine itself, for the science behind it, and for society as a whole. We'll examine some of these consequences now.

The Economics of Frontier Medicine

Like their counterparts in telecommunications, the only other current growth industry of comparable size, the pharmaceutical and hospital companies are preparing for the future with a round of mergers. Among the pharmaceuticals (often called pharmas in industry jargon), in 1999, Pharmacia/Upjohn bought Monsanto/Searle. This deal put two former drug competitors on the same side, which weakens the clout of consumers; it softens the financial effect of consumer backlash against Monsanto's aggressive tactics in selling its bioengineered products abroad (discussed in detail in Chapter 10); and it means that Monsanto's agrichemical know-how will be plugged in to the drug-making business. The same year, American Home Products tried to ingest Warner-Lambert but lost in court to a rival suitor, Pfizer. Then, in 2000, the biggest pharma, Glaxo-Wellcome, and number two, Schering-Plough, announced their union. The resulting conglomerate then absorbed SmithKline, and at last report Glaxo-SmithKline was about to wed American Home Products.

Thanks to these mergers, the technically demanding but enormously lucrative pharmaceutical industry is being concentrated into fewer and fewer hands, who aim to control its market from demand to supply. And oh, what demand! In 1999 the world spent $310 billion on pharmaceuticals. That amount is rising by 8 percent a year, and lately the *rate* of increase has been going up by a percentage point or two every year. In the United States, the current rate of increase in drug prices is 15 percent per year, and this seems likely to grow still further as biochemists keep adding to the drug armamentarium. The Food and Drug Administration approved 370 new drugs in the 1990s, 50 percent more than in the previous decade.

Each time two of the corporate giants in health care coalesce, the costs associated with finalizing the deal have to be folded into the prices of the resultant company's products. The acquiring company buys a majority of the selling company's stock shares. Generally it also buys factories and other physical assets, as well as the seller's important patents and licenses. Often the intangibles are priced way above current market value in anticipation of future earnings. Optimism usually drives the buyer's stock price and dividend rate higher, too. All that money flows from the customers of the new merged entity to investors of both the new and the old company. The managers of both typically get generous bonuses for negotiating the deal. They hope that much of the cost will be offset by economies of scale, diminished competition, and layoffs. The financial institutions and attorneys that do the legal and financial fixing also are handsomely rewarded. In the end, it is consumers who pay for corporate savings from monopolization and lost jobs. Investor profits and consumer losses are greatest in a high-tech, patent-driven industry where there are only a few companies selling products in each product category.

Therapeutic breakthroughs will raise the stakes even more. Many of the new technologies will give rise to entire new industries—massive opportunities for profit as well as huge new cost centers for an economy that is already spending record sums on health care.

Consider a few examples of the commercial prospects for artificial body parts and patches that loom before us.

The Food and Drug Administration approved the first artificial skin in 1998. The price started out at $1,000 per square-inch patch. Better production methods will lower that figure, but at the same time, improvements in the product will brake the price decline. Let's be optimistic and assume an average price of $250 per square inch over the next several years. Demand for the product will begin with the 600,000 Americans every year who have skin tumors removed, another 600,000 who seek treatment for diabetic ulcers, and 10,000 to 15,000 who have severe burns. Since burn victims often require large grafts, we'll posit medical requirements for at least 1.5 million square inches of skin. That's a domestic market of $375 million per year, not counting treatment for other conditions or elective cosmetic procedures.

Artificial replacements for two vital organs are on the near horizon. The first semi-artificial organ to be created for human implantation, the liver, will have immediate potential sales of 30,000. That's how many Americans die of liver failure each year. Transplants from organ donors yield only a tiny fraction of that number at present. A maker of long-lasting, fully functional new hearts at a marketable price could sell 100,000 per annum. Today's woefully inadequate designs cost $25,000 to $50,000 each. At a median figure of $37,500, makers of bioengineered replacements for these two vital organs could do about $5 billion of business every year.

Next consider what we might call socially induced illnesses, such as obesity. By the admittedly crude body-mass index tables compiled by the National Institutes of Health, more than half of all Americans are overweight (that is, 20 percent heavier than "normal" weight), and a fifth are obese (that is, 50 percent heavier).

This health problem is worst among the poorest members of

our society—black and Hispanic women, who often must satisfy their hungers on a diet too high in cheap starches. This also happens to be the economic segment to which the worst-quality food is marketed most aggressively, but that's only a difference in degree. All of us are subject to a daily barrage of seduction from vendors of fattening comfort foods, which until less than a hundred years ago—to our genes, just the blink of an eye—were luxuries even to the rich. Entire new classes of denutrified industrial foods leave our thickening bodies paradoxically undernourished, driving millions to seek the missing sustenance in . . . more food.

Result: a market for obesity treatments that starts at 125 million Americans, many of whom will try *anything* to regain control of their lipocytes. Each year they now spend over $100 billion on medical and over-the-counter weight-loss methods, none of them reliable. The whole amount is basically a huge piñata waiting for an effective treatment to break it open. Add in the demand from related maladies—hypertension, diabetes, arteriosclerosis, a poker hand of cancers—and you have some very impressive medical expenditures. Look for food conglomerates to form partnerships with drug makers so as to "serve" both ends of the market, just as Big Tobacco seeks first to addict smokers and then sell them cures for their addiction.

Obesity is only one example of so-called lifestyle diseases that await medical cures in lieu of social restructuring to minimize root causes. Others include lung diseases from smoking and air pollution, digestive and intestinal maladies from lack of enzymes and fiber in processed food, vision defects from day-long close focusing in dim schools and offices, and cardiac problems from sedentary jobs and entertainments. These and others give medical inventors a chance for handsome profits but present us all with costs that aren't so pretty.

The Cost Balloon

By its allure to all concerned, genomic medicine will accelerate not only the rise in total spending but also its rate of increase. In 1970, Americans spent $204 per capita on medicine. At an average 5 percent rate of inflation per year across the whole economy, in 2000 we should have been paying $882 per capita. The actual figure was $4,100, an increase equivalent to 11 percent per year. Even if, against all odds, the rate of increase in medical spending stays what it is now, the figure will be $82,000 per person in 2030. Assuming a population of 500 million, that's a total of $41 trillion, four times the size of our entire national economy today. If the rate of increase itself were to increase as in the past, those totals will be roughly $500,000 per year individually and $250 trillion collectively. There are no economists optimistic enough to predict a GDP able to absorb those numbers.

Of course, any dramatic change blindly extrapolated will produce startling forecasts that are unlikely to play out in reality. We're not predicting that U.S. health care in 2030 will actually cost $250 trillion. But we are saying that the recent rate of growth in health-care costs is unsustainable. What can be done to rein it in?

We cannot hope to slow that growth by law. Most of it will occur in the private sector, not in the tax-supported programs. Nor can we look to the cost-controlling power of large-scale purchasing groups for help. HMOs may have restrained costs by 2 or 3 percent of GDP over the last three decades, but even that's debatable. Some analysts think they actually have increased costs by adding a new institutional layer between patient and doctor. Future cost-control efforts by legislative fiat or by HMOs might yield a slight braking effect, but neither will derail the juggernaut.

There are at least two more factors that will help drive medical costs higher faster in the next few decades: genetic royalties and venture-capital returns. We'll discuss the former in Chapter 5. Here, we'll consider the effects of the latter.

At the beginning of the 1980s, the health-care industry attracted less than 10 percent of all venture capital in the country. Today that figure is at least 25 percent and probably over 30 percent. Estimates of the total size of the American venture-capital pie vary from $400 billion to $800 billion annually. Since not all risk capital shows up in such surveys, we'll use the higher figure in the calculations that follow.

Let's say one fourth, or $200 billion, of venture capital is invested in medicine, and the rate of return is 30 percent per year. That's about average for risk capital after you subtract the washouts. Health care must cover the investment and pay the dividend. Thus a total of $260 billion is extracted from customer payments off the top, not counting profits for the providers themselves.

Risk capital is like a river at flood tide. There are individual losers and winners, abandoned dry channels and new waterfalls. But overall the flood will pour into whatever economic sector is most inviting. No industry attracts that kind of money without near-certain long-term growth.

But doesn't the dot.com debacle of 2000 prove that venture capital was wrong about the Internet business? Might it not be wrong about the growth of medicine, too?

Possibly, but we doubt it. First of all, the Internet is a brand-new industry, and most of the failures were new companies. There weren't many giants ready to absorb the struggling small-fry. Medicine is an established industry with many large corporations eager to buy up new methods and products whose prototypes have been developed by start-ups. Furthermore, medicine has always outperformed the rest of the economy during both expansion and recession. Within it, although not all vendors or approaches succeed, nearly every new technology as a whole makes money. Thus, the enormous rate of venture-capital investment in health care is a strong predictor of the growth of medicine to one fourth, perhaps even one third, of our economy during the next 20 or 30 years.

What will spending this much of our riches on health care do to us?

Our current health-care system charges high prices that include a hefty, often outrageous profit, but it does so deceptively. Seldom are the full costs direct and recognizable. Instead, they're passed along to consumers in the form of taxes and insurance premiums, take-home wages that rise much more slowly than they otherwise would if companies weren't paying enormous insurance premiums for their employees, and decreases in public services as money is siphoned away from mass transit, for example, and into health care. The price of medical plans for large corporations rose 7.8 percent per year throughout the nineties, and it's not unusual for small companies to be driven out of business by sudden hikes of 50 percent. Yearly inflation in prescription plans is even higher: 12 percent for workers, 16 percent for retirees.

Thus, the growth of medical expenses raises prices and lowers wages. Medicine's ghostly hand hikes the phone bill, the grocery bill, the mortgage payment, and the cost of heating oil. It means that any product Americans make starts out at a 5 or 10 percent disadvantage in the global market, compared to a similar product made in a country with more cost-effective health care.

This is just one social cost of our overreliance on cost-inflated, commercialized health care. At 18 percent of GDP, it's like paying your income tax twice. This is the kind of out-of-control growth a cancer specialist would recognize. It's a pity, because given the chance to consider the individual purchases masked behind their medical-insurance contracts, people might choose to skip many of them. Instead, they sign up for yet another test, procedure, or prescription, figuring, "I'm paying for the insurance. I might as well use it."

Retail for Caste

Direct buying of health care *is* becoming more prevalent, but not in a way that most people like. In response to rising insurance prices, retail (pay-as-you-go) medicine is returning. Whether or not they can afford insurance, more and more people are paying routine medical costs out of their own pockets. Some maintain that this market force will keep medical costs from rising as fast as we fear and thus will also restrain helter-skelter innovation.

The new retail medicine is coming to dominate the midlevel market, where employee plans, getting swamped in the wake of speedboating costs, are covering less or are being phased out altogether. Insurers are dramatically raising subscribers' co-payments for expensive drugs and tests, and will continue to do so as treatment rosters expand to many times their current size. As a result, *defined contributions* will replace defined benefits in employee plans. This means that employers will put X number of dollars into an employee's medical account, rather than spelling out what treatments are covered. Once the employee empties the account, she's on her own. This isn't really insurance at all, but merely a medical savings account administered by the employer. Such plans will represent 30 to 40 percent of all medical purchasing by 2002.

For the lower-middle and working classes, this out-of-pocket medicine is basically empty-pocket medicine. Health insurance rates for families rose 8 to 20 percent per year during the late nineties, mostly because more patients are taking more drugs, and more expensive drugs, than ever before. As a result, many of those who are still insured have been forced to raise their deductibles in order to bring the premium down to an affordable range—to the point where they actually pay for all medical services directly, using the policy only as a backstop against overwhelming catastrophe.

The new retail medicine will flourish mightily not only at the low to middle levels but also at the high end in the coming decades, as genetic enhancements entice clients with large disposable incomes. The doctors of Brentwood and Palm Beach don't need to bother with insurance-policy patients.

Retail medicine's proponents argue: If those who can (or can't) afford it choose to spend their money on medical care, that's their business, isn't it? But in the end, who really pays?

Consider this: Every additional percentage point of GDP that we as a society spend on medicine is $100 billion that we can't spend on schools, the environment, child care, leisure, drug rehab, or Social Security. These foregone options are known to economists as "opportunity costs"—the costs of roads that cannot be taken, or built. These are ways we could enhance everyone's health, but we can't do so because the money is tied up in high-end medicine for the few.

We all know that the rich enjoy special access to new treatments. For example, human growth hormone injections were developed for children afflicted with dwarfism, and they quickly became available for short rich kids at $30,000 to $150,000 a year. Genentech did give its product free to some severely growth hormone–deficient children of the uninsured, but children from slightly better-off families who were members of HMOs were routinely denied treatment under HMO clauses that exclude injectibles or cosmetic procedures. Now biosynthesis is bringing the price of these hormones down, and they are entering the upper-middle-class adult rejuvenation market, while the insurance-dependent working poor are still left out.

The hospital association VHA Inc. and the health-care consulting division of Deloitte & Touche recently collaborated to produce a medical preview of the next decade, called *Health Care 2000*. They foresee a continuous upward price curve driven by avid demand for complex, rapidly evolving technology. Insurers will balk at covering many of the new treatments for all but their premium policyholders. Even after the first few years, the report concludes, most of the advances probably will be available only to the upper middle class as part of the burgeoning new retail medicine.

In the long run, the most socially damaging effect of the new retail may be the way it reinforces itself. It magnifies the economic disparities that force us to pass up other opportunities for social spending. In other words, it helps to enrich the rich and impoverish the poor, further stratifying health care by income.

Breathtaking treatments on the evening news and age-defying makeovers for celebrities will distract our attention from the fact that those below a certain upper-middle economic level will not be getting tickets to the show. The latest enhancements will not be offered in their neighborhoods. And in many neighborhoods, there will be less medicine altogether. As our total outlay for health care rises, so does infant mortality in the inner cities—one of the best measures of medical inequity.

The money to be made in expanding high-tech specialties will distort the supply side of medicine even more, by accelerating the migration of doctors away from the negative financial pole of family practice and toward the positive charge of luxury procedures. After all, doctors' incomes relative to expenses, and relative to those of other highly trained professionals—lawyers, airline pilots, HMO managers, to name a few—have been declining for many years, and their autonomy in treating the truly sick has disappeared so completely as a result of the hegemony of HMOs and their bean counting that the AMA now endorses the idea of a physicians' union.

The Drug Gap

The new retail will force agonizing decisions upon people of the lower-middle class. We can see the pressure in IRS statistics for medical deductions. In recent years, the percentage of taxpayers claiming medical deductions—that is, those who could devote more than 7.5 percent of their income to medicine not covered by insurance—has been falling. Nevertheless, the total of all medical deductions claimed has been rising. Those with more disposable income are spending more of it on medicine.

Today, the hardships stem largely from drug prices. As recently as the mid-1990s, drugs made up only 7 or 8 percent of costs in a typical health plan. Today that figure is often as high as 25 percent. It will keep climbing, too. Payers are doing their best to draw back from covering the parade of new pharmaceuticals but will be unable to resist their subscribers' demand for them completely. That demand has a real and legitimate component, but it will be enormously inflated by advertising, the single largest driver of steep increases in spending on drugs in the late nineties.

Medicare's noncoverage of drugs used to be a small hole in the safety net. Now the most commonly prescribed drugs for hypertension, depression, and cholesterol control cost $50 to $100 a month. Treatment with Pharmacia/Upjohn's Zyvox, a new antibiotic, may run $200 per day for a week or more. An elderly couple's drug bill can easily top $500 a month, and pharmaceuticals often cost more over time than do doctors and hospitals. A record 17.4 percent jump in drug prices during 1999 led legislators to introduce bills in Congress to add some coverage to Medicare, one of which might be law by the time you read this, but it's unlikely to make up even half of the shortfall. Suddenly the elderly, or their families, must choose between the blood-pressure medication and the rent. Does Granddad get the new cholesterol-control drug, or does daughter spend summer at camp learning to program a computer?

These kinds of decisions will get tougher for everyone, not only for the elderly. Pharmaceutical benefits are unlikely to keep pace with prices, either for the aged or the young. More and more, whether to purchase desired medications will become lonely individual choices for the unrich.

During the nineties, drug price increases were fairly well absorbed by family and employee plans, but fast-rising co-payments suggest that the limit has been reached. HMOs and insurers, unable to lower costs and pressured by lawsuits not to deny care, yet still bound to deliver their stockholders fresh dividends, are in no position to be generous. As prices overwhelm the state prescription-assistance programs, such as those for uninsured AIDS patients, public administrators are demanding discounts and threatening price controls, as occurred recently in California, Massachusetts, Vermont, and Maine.

Drug companies, tooling up for the new age of genomic drug making, will continue to resist price-controlling efforts with their awesome lobbying firepower. They are, after all, in the catbird seat, with plenty of cash to woo legislators: The top ten pharmaceutical companies report profits around 30 percent, and the industry as a whole averages 18.6 percent, nearly 3 percentage points above banking.

These margins should be no surprise. The federal government supplies much of the pharmaceutical companies' basic research for free, then grants them tax deductions for their own research and for marketing expenses. The latter often eat up as much as one third of total revenue, partly or wholly untaxed on the theory that it has educational content.

It's hard to rationalize such largesse as serving the public interest. As Marcia Angell, a former editor of the *New England Journal of Medicine*, observed, "To rely on the drug companies for unbiased evaluations of their products makes about as much sense as relying on beer companies to teach us about alcoholism." (She felt free to speak her mind in the last editorial she wrote before she resigned, on June 22, 2000.)

As prices rise, the poor will bear the brunt of the changes. And, according to the 1998 United Nations *Human Development Report*, they constitute a larger percentage of the U.S. population than that of any other major industrialized nation. The 45 million Americans with no medical insurance constitute a reservoir of aspiring demand, which can be used to sop up some subsidized care but can also be jettisoned when financial seas turn choppy— bodies in the bank, so to speak.

Recently this reserve demand has been growing by 4 or 5 percent, or 2 million "uncovered lives," per year. The 1996 welfare cutbacks added 3 million to the total, more than half of them children, when they lost benefits from Medicaid (the federal health program for welfare recipients). The federal government provides $500 million annually to the states to pick up some of the slack, but most of this goes unused as states seek to trim their Medicaid matching payments. The uninsured total does not include 20 million elderly Americans who have no drug coverage. Without a change in the law, *that* total may as much as double after Baby Boomers start retiring in 2010. Pharmaceutical prices will also *at least* double, and probably double again, by 2015.

Meanwhile, Medicare clients, the working and nonworking elderly, are being unloaded from the program–a practice often called dumping–by HMOs who took over portions of Medicare caseloads but now look for any pretext to rid themselves of the sick. Now, the term "redumping" is being added to our stock of jargon. (See the next chapter for more on this topic.) Dumping saves money for HMOs and insurers, but it costs society a lot more when the dumpees get sick enough for the emergency room, or lose their jobs and savings to ill health.

If the recent past is an indicator of the future, the drug gap will show frontier medicine at its worst. Hundreds of thousands, even millions, of people will be dying each year while the treatments that would save them are unreachable behind the plate glass windows of the Medical Boutique.

Eventually our response (or nonresponse) to the medically homeless will show what kind of society we are. Underlying the specific issues is a more general question: Is health care a right or a commodity?

CHAPTER 4

Market
über Alles

IN THE PREVIOUS TWO CHAPTERS, we have examined the roots of our insatiable appetite for health care and its side effects in terms of sheer cost. Now we're in a position to predict how the new medicine will evolve in a world increasingly ruled by market forces, where patients are seen more as consumers than as the sick needing care.

Bottom-Line Health Care

Shopping skills will become more important in the consumer-driven medicine of the future. It will be mostly up to the individual to find the right products and avoid the lemons, just as in buying a car. The difference is that with a car, barring a fatal malfunction, the consumer can eventually buy another one. Genetic modification will usually be more lasting.

Advertising will play as large a role in consumer medicine as it does in other consumer markets. In fact, the infiltration of hucksterism into medicine is already far advanced. A recent study has shown that an astounding 80 percent of educational health-care material for both the general public *and for doctors* is produced or subsidized, in whole or in part, by the pharmaceutical companies. And that's not counting direct-to-consumer advertising. When you add that in, the figure may be closer to 95 percent! Self-health books from small publishers represent one of the few outlets for health information not funded by medical corporations.

Of course, advertising technology will evolve along with medicine. The line between entertainment and marketing has been blurred for a long time, and the line between infomercials and medical reporting seems to be getting fuzzier, too. Moreover, virtual-reality engineers are rapidly erasing the boundary between media and life itself.

When you can escape your life to star in your favorite movie into which promos have been seamlessly woven, how will you even *see* the ads, much less resist them? In 25 years, it might be feasible to engineer into the vat-grown white meat you consume the genes for a drug that will induce in you a "buy" response to subliminal cues embedded in a Web-surround commercial—at the least a believe-the-message emotion and perhaps even a brand-name purchase action. In 50 years, when some superagency delivers its message digitized in proteins dissolved in your mouthwash, along with playback triggers to upload them into memory, how will you spit it out?

As medicine shifts its emphasis from therapy to upgrades, it will rely more heavily on advertising, for the same reason that other industries do: In an affluent empire that depends upon constant economic expansion, there's more money to be made in luxuries than necessities.

So medicine will have to exploit its "New! Improved!" selling points and play upon our cultural weaknesses to get us to buy more of it. Simultaneously, however, to maximize profits, commercial providers also must seek to dispense *less* medicine. That is, they have to avoid as much break-even or subsidy business with the poor as they possibly can in favor of high-end commerce.

Yet the goal of all true physicians always has been the opposite on both counts. First, they have sought to reduce demand—that is, to help customers attain long periods of trouble-free good health. For this reason, by ancient custom, Chinese doctors got paid only so long as their clients remained well. Second, as far as possible, traditional doctors *never* withheld care from the indigent, absorbing the loss or looking to their share of full-price patients to make up the difference.

Thus, the conversion of Western medicine into a for-profit industry has forced it to work against itself. It now has two primary aims: to make money for its owners and to reduce the number and needs of its customers. These aims cannot peacefully coexist. Only the stronger one will be fully served, and right now that is the corporate bottom line, not the patient's lifeline. As long as this fundamental contradiction remains, no amount of policy twiddling will ever fix our health-care system.

The commercial imperative means that in biotech medicine, whatever *can* be done *will* be done, as long as there's a paying market for it. There are no necessary bounds of taste, propriety, reverence, mercy, or simple caution in the face of our possibly incomplete knowledge—except to the extent that such considerations by individual managers and aggregated customers may affect business practice. These tempering forces are not built into the system, however, and cannot thoroughly control it. If a large conservative firm with an image to protect decides not to offer a certain outlandish option, sooner or later it will be offered by an upstart ready to gamble. Profitable damage to earth or its denizens often will be concealed rather than curtailed.

By the same token, what should be done won't be done if it's not profitable or publicly subsidized. And if it might reduce the wealth of campaign donors, it stands a poor chance of being supported by governmental subsidy.

There are many benefits we'll miss as a result. Here's just one: No pharmaceutical company will ever undertake research on herbal medicine, because the herbs cannot be patented. Finding leads toward new drugs by appropriating without compensation the age-old knowledge accumulated by vanishing aborigines, yes. Synthetic versions of the phytochemicals, yes. Expensively modified genetic products derived from plants, by all means. But applying the scientific method to update traditional use of the co-evolved bounty that grows all around us for free? Nothing could interest a capitalist less. As at present, such work will be done only on a small scale by underendowed universities and niche-market mail-order companies, typically in Canada, Scandinavia, and India. This is not to say that no one will be making money, even profiteering, on herbs and other natural remedies, just as on bottled water. The difference is in the size of the industry and the research investment behind it.

It would hardly be possible to turn back the clock, even if that offered a plausible solution. Still, the contrast between the old and the new shows what medicine has lost in the transition.

The pay-as-you-go, fee-for-service medicine of half a century ago was true retail, in the sense that there were no wholesale transactions or middlemen. Doctors and hospitals wanted to make a profit, and did, but their financial burden on society was light. There was no alternative health industry and little direct competition between hospitals or medical practices serving the same area. In most industries, lack of competition raises prices, but at that time, before widespread medical insurance coverage and elective treatments, medicine was avoided until it was unavoidable. Demand was finite.

Then, too, medicine was still mission-oriented, patient-centered. Most doctors went into the profession to help people—to make a good living, yes, but also to work long hours and receive the intangible rewards of easing people's suffering and saving their lives. During the Golden Age of American Medicine, roughly 1945 to 1965, a wave of advances—antibiotics, tranquilizers, new surgical techniques, the polio vaccines, and so on—brought an excitement to medical service that earlier and later generations of physicians have seldom known. For the first time in history, the doctor could usually take an active role, rather than being limited to offering pain relief and bedside encouragement. This was the last period in which primary-care physicians routinely made house calls—an indication of true consumer orientation.

By contrast, today's HMO medicine is pseudo-retail, because

it's profoundly antipatient. The rise of employee benefit plans has made customers an incidental annoyance, cutting them out of the decision-making loop. The bargaining is between insurer and employer, neither of whom has the potential patient's needs at heart. That's why they call it *health* insurance, as the quip goes: It stops when you get sick.

This conflict of interest—the existence of financial incentives to doctors for delaying and denying care—has sometimes come under legal challenge. Consider the case of Cynthia Herdrich, an Illinois woman who had an attack of appendicitis way back in 1991. Because she was classified as a nonemergency case, cost-saving rules imposed by her HMO, Carle Clinic Association, a division of Urbana Health Alliance Medical Plans, made her wait eight days for an ultrasound scan, a delay embodying the institutional hope that she might just go away in the meantime. Her appendix burst, however, causing her to need dangerous emergency surgery and incur *more* medical bills than if the HMO had just given her the scan when she needed it.

Ms. Herdrich sued under a clause in the 1974 Employee Retirement Income Security Act (ERISA), which requires that physicians hired by employee and retiree health plans act "solely in the interest of the participants." (That's legalese for a part of the Hippocratic oath.) Herdrich won at first, but the HMO appealed the decision, and the case went to the Supreme Court. The Court unanimously ruled that profit is the central principle of for-profit HMOs and that Congress intended it to take precedence over patient care. In his opinion, Justice David Souter said the Court "would be acting contrary to the congressional policy of allowing HMO organizations if it were to entertain [a claim] portending wholesale attacks on existing HMOs solely because of their structure."

In the new for-profit medicine, even doctors are mere extras. Many still work absurdly long hours but see only a blur of patients whisked in and out on a conveyor belt of 10-minute appointments, which the doctors may be punished for lengthening. They spend half-days on the paperwork, while patients with questions get lost in voice-mail limbo. They're pressured by management to generate simultaneously more billings and fewer treatments, and then they're second-guessed by insurers who umpire their choices from a list of recommended procedures. Thus, when a survivor of the Columbine High School massacre, Mark Taylor, after undergoing four operations, was told by his doctor that he needed an $1,800 therapeutic mattress, his HMO refused, overruling the physician.

In the mid-nineties, HMOs were severely criticized for routinely limiting new mothers and their infants to a twenty-four-hour hospital stay regardless of their condition. The practice crystallized the image of the coldheartedness of modern health care in the public's mind.

Patients' sense of impotence and betrayal emerges in jokes, like the one in which a doctor, a nurse, and an HMO director are seeking admittance to heaven. The doctor says, "I've devoted my life to the sick and have healed thousands of poor people." St. Peter waves him through. The nurse says, "I've supported the good doctor and his patients all my adult life." The gates open for her. Then the HMO director says, "I gave millions of people the most efficient care possible." St. Peter says, "Go on in. But you can only stay overnight."

Some physicians are fighting to regain control of their profession. In San Francisco and Boston, for example, hospital personnel refused to comply with government orders against treating unregistered immigrants. North Carolina doctors overwhelmed by insurance-company paperwork revolted by returning lengthy forms with only a line of dadaist comment–"The body is clean," or some such. When one psychotic patient was denied hospital time, her psychiatrist got coverage for her hospitalization by threatening to send her over to the corporate offices.

Since most states prohibit patients from suing HMOs, other doctors are trying to use malpractice law to goad medical licensers into holding HMO case reviewers to the same standards as physicians. Some state boards have been receptive, so theoretically we might see a few HMOs banned from practicing in certain states. However, the effort suffered a setback in September 2000, when Judge Barbara M. G. Lynn of the United States District Court in Dallas ruled that HMO directors are not practicing medicine but rather making coverage decisions. ERISA bars suits about such decisions.

Although advocates of unrestrained capitalism often decry the inefficiency of the public sector, the short-term expediency of business often leads to greater inefficiency in the long run. Recent attempts to reform Medicare provide a good example.

The free market was supposed to streamline the wasteful public program by administering no-frills medicine like a no-nonsense company. HMOs gladly recruited Medicare recipients in return for government bonuses. When they realized that, being old, the elderly need unpredictably large and unprofitable amounts of medicine, the companies simultaneously asked for rate increases and the right to "fire" their sickest patients like incompetent employees.

In 1998, Congress agreed that the burden of the most expensive cases should be shouldered by taxpayers, not HMOs or their investors. In the next two years, HMOs dumped 2 million of their

Medicare subscribers, about one sixth of the total. The dumping still continues today, though often indirectly. Aetna, for example, dumped about 2 million customers out of 19 million covered by its Prudential Health Care division, by means of 13 percent price hikes announced in December 2000. More than 300,000 of those were Medicare enrollees and simply could not afford the increases. The right to nullify a contract that turns out to be unprofitable, as Congress allowed HMOs to do, is seldom granted to individual taxpayers.

Medicare dumping is one variant of insurance companies' cherry picking—signing up only the young, healthy, and well employed. That's what produced managed care's lush profits early on, in the late 1980s and early 1990s. But cherries are a temperamental crop. That's the trouble with the managed-care *business*. No matter how robust your subscribers, sooner or later some of them are going to get sick. Or have accidents. Or suffer early, lingering, and expensive deaths. Or be married to someone so unfortunate. Then it will be your duty as a for-profit managed carer not to care, but instead to hustle your clients out one exit or the other with as few stops as possible along the way. No wonder HMOs are the only institutional group to achieve a lower public-confidence rating than Congress.

In the end, though, despite the suffering and deaths from wrongheaded cost control, we will be making a mistake if we focus too harshly on the "soulless managers," even the most venal. They're just being good capitalists, doing what all good capitalists must do: make money at (virtually) any cost. It's not entirely their fault that consumer concerns (What's best for the patient?) have yielded, not only in their industry but everywhere, to commercial ones (What's better for us?).

The Backlash Against HMOs

It may be that the era of the most spectacular HMO abuses has already ended. States that recently have begun to track denial-of-coverage appeals have found a surprisingly low rate of them—a little more than 1 per 500 patients in New York, for example. Perhaps the most zealous cost cutters have retreated in the face of publicity given to the horror stories. On the other hand, maybe patients have merely developed a sense of futility.

Some of the anger has borne fruit, however. In 1998, as Congress was letting HMOs off the Medicare hook, public outcry resulted in enactment of the Nevada Patient's Bill of Rights. Perhaps the most important provisions of this landmark act were those that sought to insulate medical decisions from monetary pressure. The law forbids

- Financial incentives to doctors for using fewer tests and services
- Retaliation against doctors who side with patients in disputes over coverage
- Sole determination of therapy or length of hospital stays by nonphysicians
- Gag clauses in doctors' contracts

Nevada's action sparked a torrent of regulatory bills in other states, and finally the proposal of several patient's rights bills in Congress. Perhaps these laws merely mask the need for deeper reform, as critics contend. Still, HMOs are scrambling to reinvent themselves in the public eye. Many are phasing out prior review (second-guessing the doctor) for most treatments.

It seems likely that the more successful HMOs, instead of crudely cutting costs by cutting coverage, will find ways to channel demand into more efficient tiers of treatment. Instead of making doctors submit to clipboard wielders, they will use their personnel to digest the enormous medical literature into reports of true value to their physicians. For their patients, they will emphasize education, self-health training, and low-cost natural remedies as a first resort for everyday ills. They will promote those checkups, such as prostate exams and Pap smears, that make a big difference, and avoid others, like treadmill tests and chest x-rays, that yield too many false positives for widespread use.

More and more, HMOs will serve as gateways, offering subscribers access to a wide range of medical options, customized insurance and payment plans, information, discounts, and transportation to medical centers. In exchange, they will broker their greatest assets, their "covered lives," as a market for advertisers and other health-care providers throughout the country. Gradually evolving, we hope, a more human face, managed care will continue to dominate medical commerce for the foreseeable future.

Thus, the current spasm of outrage against HMOs is forcing them to live up to some of the comforting phrases in their glossy brochures. Laws have been passed, and more will be passed, to protect people from the too-flagrant predators. Yet no matter how sweet the smile on the face of the medical marketers, the economic reality of health care seems destined to grow harsher. The industries built around food, metals, oil, vehicles, weaponry, electronics, and entertainment all bred ruthlessly exploitative competition in their early, Wild West phase. There is no reason to expect that biotechnological medicine will be any different.

CHAPTER 5

A Patent Misunderstanding

ONE MIGHT TRACE THE ORIGINS OF biotechnology as far back as 8,000 years ago, to the first use of yeast to make bread and beer, or even earlier, to the selection of desirable traits in wild grain for farming and in wild animals for breeding. But the modern era of biotechnology as science began in 1973, when the geneticists Stanley Cohen of Stanford University and Herbert Boyer of the University of California at San

Francisco discovered how to use chemicals known as restriction enzymes and ligases to cut and paste lengths of DNA. As an industry, biotechnology is even younger. It was born in 1980 out of a five–four Supreme Court decision in a dispute between a geneticist, Ananda Mohan Chakrabarty, and the U.S. Patents and Trademarks Office.

Working for General Electric, Chakrabarty had created the first genetically engineered life form, a petroleum-eating bacterium later licensed to Exxon to help clean up oil spills. But the PTO had refused to issue a patent for a living organism. The Supreme Court ruled that microorganisms *were* patentable, and Chakrabarty received his patent, but the Court requested guidance from Congress on the issue of patenting other life forms.

That guidance never came.

As a result of Congress's inaction, the gene and protein components of all life on earth have become, in the eyes of American law, a vast pool of potentially proprietary commodities no different from plastics or lasers. Not unlike the free licensing of the airwaves to for-profit broadcasters, this was a giveaway to the private sector, supposedly inadvertent, yet total. Now the grant may be impossible to rescind, although battles to limit its scope will keep many lawyers busy in the coming years.

In 1993, on the basis of genetic material in one blood sample taken from one woman, two Americans tried to patent the genome of the Guaymí tribe of Panama, which would have given them a monopoly on the biochemical basis of Guaymí resistance to certain viruses. The patent was refused by the PTO. In 1988, Baylor University applied for a European patent on human females genetically modified to produce designer drugs in their breast milk. They didn't get the patent, but their attempt raised the specter of poverty-stricken "pharm women" hiring themselves out as biofactories. Unless the legal climate changes, these foretell equally surreal but more carefully written applications that will be accepted.

In their written opinions and decisions, judges and patent examiners often seem to have been misled by a false analogy to mining. As a result, instead of merely granting genetic prospectors the right to work a land claim, they let them patent the gold itself.

Nearly all genetic entrepreneurs argue that gene patents are the only way to underwrite the long, expensive research needed to reap eventual benefits from basic knowledge. At first blush they appear to have a point. Wouldn't insulin be much scarcer and more expensive if Genentech didn't have a patent on the gene for it? The patent enabled the company to develop a bioengineered product, which lowered the price of insulin dramatically below previous methods of producing it.

But when applied to all genetic research, could that argument be a rationalization after the fact? Perhaps a national debate, of the kind that briefly flourished amid the 1993 health-care reform effort, could have yielded a tax-supported research program of adequate scope and speed, balanced by people's desire for nonmonetary values in their medicine. Perhaps making life a patent-free zone would have slowed the advent of novel technologies to a less dangerous pace, allowing more thoughtful public control of the process.

Furthermore, a distinction needs to be made between a *method* and genetic material itself. Patents on a method for using a certain DNA sequence to make an organism for a specific commercial purpose, if such procedural patents were clearly distinguished from patents on the life form itself, might actually nourish invention better. By keeping the genetic code free, they would encourage diverse approaches to each problem instead of limiting a genetic sector of inquiry to one patent holder, the first prospector to stake a claim.

The contrast between today's medicine and that of fifty years ago is striking. When Edward R. Murrow asked Jonas Salk, the developer of the first polio vaccine, who would own his vaccine, he replied, "Well, the people, I would say. There is no patent. Could you patent the sun?"

It may already be too late to reverse the momentum of genetic ownership. The court created a gold rush, and now we have to play by gold rush rules. The Human Genome Project was one of the first mad stampedes inspired by the frontier atmosphere.

The 50,000-Gene Dash

The Human Genome Project was virtually unheralded when its founding director, James Watson, with Francis Crick one of the original discoverers of the structure of DNA, began it in 1985 as a projected 20-year endeavor. Watson organized a group of university labs, for the most part publicly funded, in the United States, Europe, and Japan, whose scientists gradually learned how to decode and piece together stretches of DNA long enough to contain entire genes. The scientists worked in the traditional way, sharing their results with each other and other interested parties. By 1997 they had deciphered the base-pair sequence of perhaps half of all human genes, but they did not yet have a way to map most of these pieces to their actual location amid the nongenetic "junk" DNA of each chromosome and so to produce a complete sequence of the entire genome end to end.

In that year, however, the situation abruptly changed, and the Human Genome Project became a spectacle of science as athletic event. It was a race—a race to market.

In 1997, J. Craig Venter announced that his Celera Corporation had a so-called "shotgun" approach to the monumental task: they were using hundreds of computers and proprietary software to assemble a map of the genome in one go, instead of the laborious piece-by-piece method pioneered by the scientists of the public consortium. In the press, Venter became the swift, modern-money hare, starting late but still running past the plodding government turtles in the human genome marathon. There was talk in Congress of abandoning the nonprofit project, and it seemed that the human genetic code would become company property of Celera.

A lesson in the superiority of the private sector? Maybe. But the situation is not so clear-cut. For one thing, the private sector generally uses tax-supported research at will while hiding its own data from tax-funded scientists. Interestingly, Venter, though called an industrial bad boy, yielded to a torrent of criticism from scientists and published much of Celera's raw data, even though other companies would comb it for their own proprietary databases of medically significant genes.

And because of Celera's challenge, the first wave of genome-based medical development will arrive at least three years sooner than it otherwise would have. This is certainly good for people whose afflictions are addressed in that interval, but the costs and benefits for society as a whole are harder to assess.

Furthermore, the mathematician Eugene W. Myers, who devised the shotgun method for sequencing whole genomes, had offered it first to the public consortium. They told him it wouldn't work, so he took it to Celera instead—who proved it would work. That's certainly a point for private initiative.

On June 26, 2000, in a news conference at the White House, President Clinton announced completion of the Human Genome Project by both teams simultaneously—in other words, neither one side nor the other was proclaimed the winner. This statement was widely interpreted as an arranged draw to save face for the government scientists. But it turned out that they had had a ninth-inning slugger, in the person of James Kent, a genetics grad student from the University of California at Santa Cruz.

By early 2000, the public consortium had mapped most of the genome in short lengths but still had no way to put the pieces together into the whole picture. Appalled at the prospect of the assembled genome sequence locked up in a corporate safe, Kent wrote assembler software for the consortium. He did what normally would be a year's worth of work for a half dozen programmers in one month of keyboarding so furious that he had to ice down the swelling in his wrists. When the two sides compared notes after the news conference, it turned out that the public sector, with Kent running the last leg of the relay, had actually beaten Celera to the full sequence by three days. Aesop's fable of the tortoise and the hare comes to mind, and there must be some kind of moral here about turning science into a sponsor-directed sport.

Certainly Kent is a hero. But over the long haul, the most valuable players from the perspective of the public interest were the British partners. Throughout the project, John E. Sulston, director of the Sanger Center near Cambridge, insisted as a condition of his participation that all data be published free on the Internet daily. The thanks of a grateful world should go also to Michael Dexter, director of the Wellcome Trust, and Dr. Michael Morgan, coordinator of the British team's financial backing via that institution. In the face of American doubts about paying to complete the seemingly lost race, Dexter and Morgan vowed that if necessary the trust would supply the funds for British scientists to finish the job alone, to ensure that a reference copy of the human genome would enter the public domain no matter what Congress or any corporation might do.

In any case, it appears that the last-minute combination of the two teams' data, from Celera's top-down method and the government's bottom-up piece-by-piece approach, have yielded a better map of the human genome than either would have done alone. Successful completion of the project gives us a letter-by-letter readout of the complete DNA of a human being. (Actually, a composite was made from several individuals by both Celera and the consortium.) Scientists now have a framework within which to fit everything they're learning about human genetics, and the entire code book in which to seek further discoveries. Over the Internet via Mr. Kent's software, it is available to all for research or viewing.

The next step is to *annotate* the genome—to try to figure out the function and location of each gene. Early in 2001, hundreds of geneticists at the world's major genetics research centers gathered electronically in a series of round-the-clock brainstorming sessions—the so-called annotation jamboree. Using DNA-pattern-matching software, they predicted the location of most of the still-unknown genes within the raw sequence, filled in the name and function of the relatively few genes already known from previous research, and made predictions based on position and nucleotide spelling about the function of many of the others. Those hypotheses will set the course of genetic research for years to come.

Meanwhile, the open-research pattern of the Human Genome Project is being applied to various follow-on projects, the majority in further competition with private companies. These are some of the most important:

- The National Institutes of Health's Mammalian Gene Collection Project is building a public library of animal genomes. It now holds data on about 75,000 species, including animals, plants, microbes, and viruses.
- Various companies will mine public sequences with their own software, organizing the data for resale to a range of customers, from individual researchers working on a shoestring to deep-pocket pharmas.
- A consortium of 10 pharmaceutical companies and five nonprofit research institutions formed to create a public database of medically important human SNPs (single nucleotide polymorphisms) finished the first phase of its work in 2001. However, suspicion that some of the drug companies raided the preliminary data for patents on the sly has led to turmoil.
- The Berkeley Drosophila Genome Project is bringing the fruit fly genome, already mapped in partnership with Celera, to the full annotation level—understanding the function of each gene.
- The National Cancer Institute's Cancer Genome Anatomy Project is working on a full sequence-and-analysis database of normal, precancerous, and cancerous cells in humans and in the animals most commonly used in cancer research.
- Epigenomics, a German company, has joined several genetics institutes in the European Union to form the

Human Epigenome Consortium (HEC). The HEC plans to map the body's 400,000 methylation switch settings. Methylation is a chemical process that turns off a gene by reversibly covering it with an inert molecule. It's the basic way that a cell regulates which of its genes are active at a given moment, and defects in a cell's methylation process can cause it to become cancerous. The academic centers intend to put the basic data in the public domain, while Epigenomics plans to create a commercial database on the differences between healthy and diseased tissue. It will license its data to makers of drugs and diagnostic tests.

- In a project nicknamed The Wall, technicians at the Harvard Medical School Institute of Proteomics are building a "seed catalogue" of all human genes, consisting of samples of each one replicated to form a substantial amount of the pure gene ready for use in medical research. But that's only the first stage. They also plan to amass a sample base of all 100,000 human proteins. The service will be free to academics and fee-based to for-profit developers.

- Myriad Genetics of Salt Lake City, in a technical and investment partnership with Hitachi, Oracle, and Friedli Corporate Finance, a Swiss investment bank, plans to compile its own proprietary human proteome database.

- Several companies are devising ways to speed up the most tedious and difficult part of proteomic analysis— determining the precise amino acid structure of proteins. Two San Diego firms, Structural GenomiX and SyrRx, the latter a subsidiary of the pharmaceutical giant Novartis, are jockeying for an early lead in solving protein structures for private and public research databases.

Despite the public-private partnerships that many of these entities have created, however, all of these projects are proceeding under the shadow of battles over private versus public control of genetic knowledge and the profits it may someday yield.

Staking Claims on the Genetic Frontier

Just as the fevered hunt for oil reserves can make geologists who just like to study rocks seem quaint, so commercial genetics obscures the very idea of a *non*commercial side. Yet many branches of science are profiting from the new understanding of DNA—in terms not of financial gain but of increase in knowledge with little commercial potential.

For example, genomics is revolutionizing the study of human history and migration. Witness the recent finding that the spread of *Homo sapiens sapiens* (earlier termed Cro-Magnon man) into Europe from the Near East occurred via just seven women. Further back, 144,000 years ago to be approximate, the entire lineage of our subspecies passed through just one ancestral Eve. Studies of the Y chromosome point to one Adam at the same time.

Closer to our own era, genetics has confirmed the validity of the oral history of the Lemba, a tribe of southern Africa, which traces their descent from an exiled lost tribe of Israel. DNA studies have even linked the Lemba clan that led the migration with modern Jewish priestly families.

Genomics might help resurrect lost species, too. A group under Mike Archer, director of the Australian Museum in Sydney, has extracted long pieces of DNA from a preserved specimen of a thylacine, the Tasmanian wolf (also called the Tasmanian tiger, but actually a marsupial), which became extinct in 1936. The team still must somehow fill in the missing genes, grow live thylacine cells, find or engineer a suitable surrogate mother animal or artificial womb, and reconstruct the beast's vanished habitat, but extracting the DNA is an exciting first step. The endeavor might even pay off in *Jurassic Park*–type tourism someday. Other scientists are working backward from modern varieties of yeast to synthesize a prehistoric common ancestor, hoping to learn how to trace the steps of evolution backward, from birds to dinosaurs.

Genome scanning may even aid literary studies on occasion. Plans are under way to try piecing together thousands of tattered fragments of the Dead Sea Scrolls using genetic tests to sort out which pieces of vellum came from the same sheep or goat. A similar process might be used to match scraps of papyrus by ascertaining which strain of *Cyperus papyrus* rush was used to make them.

When compared to the vast amounts of money and work being invested in genetic products, efforts such as these sometimes seem like mere furtive whispers from an alley meandering off the Great Gold Way. Still, they remind us that we live not by bread alone. Certainly the men freed by genetic testing after being wrongly imprisoned for rape and murder would agree to the value of noncommercial genetic research.

Depositing the complete human genome sequence in the public domain may prevent some problems that otherwise might arise from private ownership of it. Much research on the whole human genome and on some cross-species comparisons will remain unfettered by patent-infringement concerns. But the rush to commercialize individual genes nonetheless threatens us with a host of potential problems, including a new cycle of medical expansion and profiteering.

A great many scientists are furious about the new confusion in patent law engendered by the Supreme Court's ruling in the Chakrabarty case. Two previously distinct legal entities have been confounded: a *discovery*, previously not patentable, and an *invention*, which has always been subject to patent protection. This confusion corrupts basic research, turning it from a cooperative quest for truth into a winner-take-all treasure hunt.

In the resulting legal climate, companies are rushing to patent human genes by structure alone, with no clue as to their function. To date, more than 1,000 human genes and about 5,000 from other organisms have been patented. In fact, many patents have been granted for expressed sequence tags (ESTs), chunks of raw code that are merely *thought* to contain genes or parts of genes. The PTO had begun limiting EST patents to very short lengths, both to increase revenue by multiplying the number of applications and to limit the practice of claiming huge tracts of genetic land for prospecting later. Now the office is phasing out EST patents. But the whole situation remains a morass of future legal problems.

We're learning that many genes have multiple functions, depending on what cell they're in, what other genes they interact with, nutritional status and age of the organism, and probably other factors not yet known. Fear of lawsuits may well prevent research even on functions of genes that the patent holder is not investigating. For example, all research on the two known BRCA (breast-cancer) genes—genes where mutations associated with breast cancer risk are known to take place—is now limited to one company, Myriad Genetics, which has already shut down a University of Pennsylvania research project on the genes by threatening a patent-infringement lawsuit. In the current legal situation, it is possible for a company to patent your own genetic idiosyncrasies, even if learned from a sample taken for other purposes, then force you to pay for using your own genes medically. A scientist might discover leads for cure of a disease involving several genes, only to be torpedoed by a "submarine patent," a company's long-ago-reserved rights to a key part of one of the genes. That company could hold the entire project hostage. Perhaps lawyers might devise a type of class action on behalf of disease victims, on the theory that inhibiting the relevant research is like withholding water from a person dying of thirst.

Patent problems extend beyond the genes, too. Because of discoveries made at the University of Wisconsin, the Wisconsin Alumni Research Foundation (WARF) happens to have patents on a half dozen of the most valuable lines of human embryonic stem cells. Wanting to make its stem cells available to all labs while ensuring a livelihood for its scientists, the alumni group had been selling the right to use the lab-grown cells for a mere $5,000 per cell line. To handle the actual licensing and sales, the group signed an agreement with Geron Corporation, giving the company intellectual property rights for use of those cell lines in medical treatments. However, Geron raised the licensing fees dramatically, and WARF is now suing the company to force it to lower the price it charges nonprofit researchers.

Legal problems in medical genetics recently became even knottier. The annotation jamboree came up with only 30,000 to 40,000 genes in the human genome, one third as many as previously estimated. This has of course shrunk the pie, sending biotech stocks into a tailspin. More important for the state of our knowledge, however, is that it also means that genes interact in networks that are much more complex than previously thought. Each patent may end up infringing on dozens or hundreds of others.

Another legal headache arises from the manner in which much research is conducted. Many researchers have multiple contracts with government agencies, universities, and corporations. Working concurrently on two or three projects, each scientist normally collaborates with other scientists in distant cities, each of whom has the same multiple ties. Several such groups study a single gene, others work on the proteins it makes, and others on the receptors, catalysts, and deactivating enzymes. All of the investigators may have valid, litigable patent claims. Legal fees to sort out these problems could be heavy.

The practice of patenting genes by structure, without knowing what they do, will also raise the cost of genetic medicine. In 2000, Human Genome Sciences Inc. (HGSI) laid claim to a mystery gene that, as other researchers found, makes the protein to which the AIDS virus bonds when it infects a human T cell. The company will be entitled to royalties on any vaccine developed to close this gateway—even without doing any work on it.

Several other companies, notably HGSI and Incyte, routinely submit patent applications for genes they find simply by scanning the public database. Though many genes may have no medical use, such prospectors reason that they can at least mass-produce the proteins made by the genes, then sell them to makers of pet and livestock feed.

The consequences of this legal limbo are grave for medical futures, in both senses of the word. Without a drastic change in the legal rules, nearly all medically exploitable genes will be privately owned by 2003. A company that wants to put together a microarray assay chip of 10,000 genes useful in screening for a wide range of cancers will have to pay a royalty on every one of them. This could make genetic testing too expensive for all but the superrich. At the very least, there will be a business niche for a service to track use of genetic material and capture biotech royalties, much as the music industry tracks songs to capture royalties.

Some pharmaceutical companies, even the giants, are having second thoughts about genetic drug design, as they're finding that paying royalties on human genes, genetically altered test mice, cell lines, and growth media can make many a drug too expensive to develop, even without the risk of being sued for patent infringement.

All of this helps explain the Wild West frenzy of the gene grab. The movie rights to a blockbuster may be precious, but think of your income if you owned the letter *e* and could demand payment anytime someone used it. Owning a gene could prove to be just that valuable.

In *The Biotech Century,* Jeremy Rifkin insightfully compared the genetic patent grab with enclosure, the legal doctrine that ownership of land is absolute and that landlords may fence off their holdings to prevent all public use thereof. In parallel with the rise of capitalism, primarily between the sixteenth and nineteenth centuries, enclosure reduced nearly every square inch of land in England and Europe to restricted private use. Most of the rest of the earth has been similarly parceled out since then. Even parks and nature preserves must be bought with tax money. There is no assumed right for them to exist or for the public to enjoy them.

Since enclosure, the largest amount of most people's time is no longer devoted to getting food or pursuing pleasure but rather to earning money with which to pay landowners for the right to occupy a space on the earth. Besides providing the basis of modern capitalism, enclosure erased from human thought the very idea of "common ground," which had underlain all societies through the medieval period.

Now gene enclosure threatens to further reduce the power of people against aggregated capital. Despite strenuous opposition by indigenous peoples throughout the world, plans go forward for the Human Genome Diversity Project, a sort of biological museum that will collect the genomes of some 750 isolated, ancient populations before they disappear. Nothing wrong with that in a wholly just world, but think what it means in ours. First World peoples who have taken natives' land and resources by force now may expropriate their DNA to be mined for patentable products that will benefit only themselves.

If completed, genetic enclosure will reduce every molecule of life on earth to private property, only this time the natives won't even get a reservation in the desert. Bioprospecting—the worldwide search for purebred strains of plant, animal, and human DNA with unique traits that can be locked up in Western patents—is laying the foundations for the twenty-first century's towers of wealth, but it also may be the aspect of biotechnology most likely to light the fires of resistance. The struggle will be won or lost on a worldwide basis. Even if a nation were to try to prevent export of indigenous species for commercial exploitation, biotech know-how can appropriate gene rights on the basis of no more than a few cuttings or tissue samples in a suitcase.

Madagascar may well become the poster child for genetic colonialism. Its varied terrain and its geologic separation from Africa have made it, in genetic terms, perhaps the richest country on earth. Economically, however, it is one of the poorest. For many years it has depended on one source of export income—the vanilla bean orchid. Now the cellular chemistry that produces the key vanilla taste protein has been reproduced in at least two laboratories. As soon as the protein's structure or that of the gene that makes it is patented, the life technology behind this flavoring, so widely used that its name has become an adjective meaning "unflavored," will be owned for production elsewhere. Of course, there will be no compensation whatsoever to the island where it evolved, nor to the 100,000 farmers who grow the crop today.

Automated biofactories portend a huge, rapid elimination of different types of work in all parts of the world. Similarly, the monetary value of all localized plant and animal products is about to disappear. Lest you think that this is only a "poor nation" problem, consider: Cotton boll cells and orange and lemon juice cells have been lab-grown in prototype techniques. Communities in Florida, California, and across the American South will suffer the eventual consequences.

Early Fiascos in Gene Therapy

In the broadest sense, gene therapy isn't completely new. Scarce hormones and drugs have been mass-produced for decades by inserting the genes for them into bacteria, beginning with insulin in 1978 and interferon in 1980. But the new gene-alteration therapy in humans, so widely and enthusiastically touted in the media, has gotten off to an absurd start. Between 1985 and the turn of the millennium, over 300 clinical trials had been conducted, and only one usable treatment had emerged—VEGF (vascular endothelial growth factor) gene injections to grow small coronary arteries. In April 2000, the cure by Dr. Alain Fischer of two French babies born with severe combined immunodeficiency syndrome (SCID) reassured us that more great things are yet to come. Still, the chief result so far has been a parade of incompetent venality that has surprised even the field's harshest critics.

Here are some examples.

On September 11, 1999, Jesse Gelsinger became the first patient known to have died from gene therapy. The Tucson teenager had volunteered to test a medicine for a rare liver-enzyme deficiency in a program at the University of Pennsylvania.

His own deficiency was mild and was well controlled by drugs, but Jesse had offered his body for a trial of the treatment on behalf of young children, in whom the malady is often fatal. The medicine's modified cold-virus vector caused an uncontrollable immune reaction, which killed the young man.

The experimenters, including the team leader, Dr. James Wilson, had behaved shamefully. They had failed to mention to their test subjects similar immune reactions encountered in trials on monkeys, as well as the fact that several members of the Recombinant DNA Advisory Committee (RAC) of the National Institutes of Health (NIH) had thought the test too risky to proceed. The experimenters also told Gelsinger and his father, Paul, that the treatment had produced a 50 percent increase in the production of the desired liver enzyme in another patient, only to admit in the post-death investigation that it had done no such thing. Furthermore, Dr. Wilson owned stock in the company, Genovo, that sponsored the tests.

Meanwhile, University of Pennsylvania officials busied themselves with producing a self-serving report on the incident, whose conclusions were completely at variance with those of the Food and Drug Administration. The FDA probe found eighteen types of improper procedures and violations of rules on reporting and informed consent. The only one to emerge from the affair with any credit was Paul Gelsinger, who, despite his terrible loss, forgave: "These guys screwed up, yes. But they should not be put out of business. They should be able to lick their wounds and go back to work. They'll be clean from now on. I want them to make this thing work, and do it right." It was a generous reaction—perhaps excessively so.

That same autumn, the National Cancer Institute of the NIH was working with researchers at Georgetown University to test a new gene drug against colon cancer. Unfortunately, they sent the wrong test medication to Georgetown. No one at either end noticed the error until it had been given to six subjects.

The mistake apparently caused the patients no harm, except for the delay involved. However, it came to light only because Representative Henry Waxman of California decided to give medical experiment reporting practices a checkup in the wake of the Gelsinger episode. At both the University of Pennsylvania and the NIH, Waxman found consistent secrecy and failure to report deaths and other adverse events in trials of genetic medicine, even events completely unrelated to the therapy.

In four frustrating months of investigation, the congressman found it "extraordinarily difficult and time-consuming" to get basic information on test outcomes. This is not a good way to win public confidence in new technology.

On June 29, 2000, the Department of Health and Human Services Office for Human Research Protection shut down 75 genetic therapy experiments at the University of Oklahoma Health Sciences Center in Tulsa for gross breaches of safety and consent norms. In one experiment, at least 100 patients with melanoma were injected with a vaccine made by untrained lab workers, which was not checked for contamination.

Worse, doctors told subjects that the shots could shrink their tumors, when in fact the vaccine was being tested in low doses for toxicity only. Nor did they warn them of the risk of forgoing other treatment to be in the nontherapeutic experiment. Twenty-six of them died during the study, but no one followed up to see whether it was the vaccine or the cancer that killed them. As the president of the Health Sciences Center, Kenneth Lackey, said after his own inquiry, "There is no excuse for what we did."

Paying more attention to medical trials after young Gelsinger's death, NIH regulators found that only 39 of 691 "serious adverse events" in human gene therapy experiments at other institutions had been reported. Common reactions included fever and sharp drops in blood pressure, typical of the immune response that killed Gelsinger. In other cases, needle damage from brain injections caused paralysis and loss of speech; three of six patients in one experiment where such techniques were used died.

In a test of VEGF injected into the heart to grow new coronary vessels, one patient died two months later, possibly as a result of the treatment. In the same study, one of the experimenters, Jeffrey Isner, and coworkers twice saw a tumor in the lung of another man, a heavy smoker, but withheld the knowledge from him and went ahead with the experiment, knowing that the growth factor might accelerate the cancer, which did in fact grow until the patient found out about it himself two months later during hospitalization for the pain. As is common these days, Isner is a leading shareholder in Vascular Genetics of Durham, North Carolina, primary sponsor of the study.

Most unnerving, perhaps, is the fact that some of the world's deadliest diseases are being tinkered with by researchers. Early in 1999, researchers began transmuting HIV-1, the AIDS virus, for use as a transport vector to get therapeutic genes into cells, possibly even for use in a kind of genetic jujitsu to turn the disease against itself. News reports featured reassurances from scientists that the work couldn't possibly infect anyone with AIDS by accident. Only a year later, experimenters at Baylor College of Medicine in Houston and St. Jude Children's Research Hospital in Memphis thought they might have infected children with live HIV and hepatitis C viruses in a batch of experimental genetic medicine that staff had overlooked when testing for contamination as per protocol. Thankfully, the scare proved to be a false alarm, and the subjects were in end-stage neuroblastoma anyway, so any error would have been moot.

But what about next time?

The Pressure to Produce at Any Cost

Market imperatives partly explain the conflicts of interest behind most of these concealments. It's often easy to get some results in petri dishes and lab animals—enough for overeager headline writers to use in stories that justify funding decisions but still far from producing a safe, decisive therapy for humans. Once a hint of future success exists, corporate interests quickly become involved. Usually the most basic research is underwritten by public agencies, but for additional funds most labs sign away rights in any eventual product to corporate backers. The lead researchers generally get stock in the company, as Dr. Wilson did in Genovo, which funded the liver-enzyme medicine tests at the University of Pennsylvania.

Often the moneymen step in at the first hint of a breakthrough and force the scientists to slap together a clinical trial (even though most academicians have never run one), hoping that the immature technique will suffice for them to cash in before somebody else does it better. It's like expecting the Wright brothers to fly their first crude plane from Kitty Hawk to London—with passengers aboard.

Personal career ambition also plays a huge role in the rush to declare research victories. Whoever invents a way to fix genetic defects permanently and reliably anywhere in the body will win the Nobel Prize and become incredibly rich and famous. In return for their life's work on the same problem, a few others who come in second or third in the great race will get, at most, a paragraph or two in some academic history of science mouldering on a library's dusty shelf. That's just how it is. Erwin Chargaff discovered the base-pair chemistry of DNA, but Watson and Crick put it all together into the double helix, so they're the only ones you've ever heard of. Doing work one loves is a tremendous privilege, of course, and one must enjoy it for its own sake or find another career. Still, no one wants to die forgotten.

The motives may be understandable, but the results are not excusable. The Stanford University geneticist Patrick Brown put it in perspective:

> Even if a scientist can prevent personal financial interests
> from corrupting decisions involving patient care, the inability
> to set aside personal enrichment for a higher good invites
> public cynicism, especially in a situation where patients are
> asked to put themselves at risk for the good of others.

In mid-2000, Health and Human Services Secretary Donna Shalala asked Congress for authority to fine those who violate the rules of experimental ethics. That would be a good first step, but it's at least as important to expand the various agencies' review boards, which are now strained beyond capacity by the huge increase in the volume and pace of research.

Our response will help determine the tenor of all genetic medicine, for we're being forced once more to decide where government shall stand between the extremes of being a sword for business and a shield for consumers. Better regulation will help, but only a change of heart within the industry can solve the problem completely.

U.S.-based biotechnology's offensive tactics already have caused much backlash abroad (see Chapter 10). If genetic medicine wants to escape being tarred with the same brush, it had better clean up its act fast.

CHAPTER 6

False Profits

MOST PREDICTIONS ARE TOO ROSY in some crucial respect. We hope for the best, and we sight into the future the only way we can, along a straight line. But new technologies usually develop as breakthroughs followed by slow consolidation, punctuated by failures. The failures rarely force a change of direction. They just add to the total price.

Early proponents of nuclear power, promising energy "too cheap to meter," attracted headlong investment and federal immunity from damage claims. Unfortunately, the costs that no one wanted to think about in the beginning—accidents, evacuation planning, mounting public distrust, waste disposal, and decommissioning scores of nuclear plants—made nuclear power "too expensive to use." Unfortunately, we were stuck with it. At least, the public was stuck with it. The original investors had already taken their gains, sticking taxpayers and public utilities with the phase-out costs.

Health on a national scale is more like renewable energy than like nuclear power. It needs long-term planning and local initiative more than short-term fixes and centralized control by giant institutions.

Will bad medicine inevitably drive out good? How much of the history of nuclear power will repeat itself in commercialized genetics? For a hint of an answer, let's consider the evolution of another high-tech industry—the computer software business.

The software industry has produced some programs that give us remarkable productivity, efficiencies, and artistic possibilities. It has also drained countless hours from the lives of millions of people struggling to use the often bug-ridden, poorly designed, and needlessly complex programs. Computer users often have to cobble together patches and work-arounds so as to get even routine jobs done. Rebooting and a trip to the water cooler have become part of the office routine. No one can guarantee that the system will work the same way two days in a row, and God help the adventurous soul who tries everything on the menu.

The Microsoft monopoly has contributed enormously to the shortfall in software quality. As the joke goes, Bill Gates once wished he had a penny for every time Windows crashed—and now he does!

Software quality will play a critical role in the medicine of the future, because only computers enable scientists to manipulate the enormous, mind-numbing stretches of repetitive code that constitute our genome. In personal-computer software, the results of corporate arrogance are somewhere between demoralizing and infuriating. Now imagine the same arrogance applied to the next huge domain for software design—genetic medicine. Bugs in the code won't be quite so funny if the Blue Screen of Death stops being a metaphor.

It would be nice to believe that software made to manage the molecular details of life will be designed with far greater diligence than are current consumer programs. So far, there's no reason to assume this will happen.

Knowledge Locked in a Vault

Monopolistic carelessness won't be the only source of problems in the genetic industry. Secrecy will be another.

Through the eighties, the federal government was the largest source of money for scientific research, particularly for basic research in pursuit of knowledge that might not lead to a product right away. Applied research and engineering, built on the fruits of public labor, were traditionally the province of industry. Each sector, public and private, spent about $60 billion to $75 billion a year.

In the mid-nineties this alignment abruptly changed. Spurred by developments in computers and biotechnology, private enterprise tripled its research-and-development budget between 1994 and 1999, while government funding stayed about the same, at $100 billion or so. The differential is much greater in the medical industry. Pharmaceutical companies devote over a fifth of their revenue to R&D, and their total, now over $26 billion, is growing by 10 percent a year. Moreover, much of the private funding does not show up in surveys, since it is devoted to a clandestine search for patentable technology. It may be stashed away in another department, at a subsidiary company, or done off the books altogether to keep the knowledge from corporate rivals. Some analysts believe that private medical-science investors soon will outspend tax-supported medical research institutions by a hundred to one.

This imbalance between publicly and privately funded research poses increasing problems in the area of secrecy. Scientists must always strike a balance between openness and stealth. They need to protect their original work until it is published, yet the advancement of knowledge cannot continue unless scientists share their results with colleagues.

Corporate control is damming this flow of information. To a large degree there is no longer one science, into whose great pool of knowledge each investigator drops her new thimbleful after a gestation period in concealment. Instead, there are now as many sciences as there are competitors in each discipline—or each market. There's a Pfizer chemistry, a Searle chemistry, a Celera genomics, an Incyte genomics, and so on, all jealously guarded, almost as separate as parallel universes.

Scientists who work in one cosmos cannot discuss their work with those in the one next door. Often they are forbidden to present preliminary findings at conferences where they would traditionally have received feedback from their peers. And if not prevented by their employer, they still know that the big-name journals won't publish a paper if any work in it has been previously reported, so they labor in isolation.

The control of knowledge by money is creating a series of related problems for the entire scientific enterprise. Consider, for example, its effects on scholarly publishing. On the one hand, the financial realities of research dictate that, of the 25,000 scientific journals published today, perhaps two thirds of them amount to clutter, printing inferior work or papers spun off from those submitted to the prestige outlets. They exist for the simple reason that no scientist can get a grant without being published. They produce a background noise in which one of the things a scientist looks for in the literature—a glimpse of someone else working on the same problem—can easily get lost.

On the other hand, the top journals have become such big businesses that many libraries can no longer afford their subscription prices, some now over $10,000 a year. Worse, their ad revenue is now so important to them that they cannot publish anything that will offend a sponsor.

Back in 1992, Dr. Suzanne W. Fletcher, then editor of *Annals of Internal Medicine,* published an article about deceptive drug advertising in medical journals. The resulting loss of $1.5 million in pharmaceutical advertising revenue cost Fletcher her job, and there have been no more articles published in that periodical on that topic. In 1999, the editors of the *New England Journal of Medicine* and the *Journal of the American Medical Association* were both forced to resign in disputes over the tailoring of content to market. As Lawrence Altman tactfully noted in reporting these two firings in the *New York Times,* "Money is changing the meaning of editorial freedom."

It gets worse. Private sector–funded research on humans completely lacks the peer reviews and test-subject safeguards required in federally funded work. As a result, development of breakthroughs is likely to be accelerated—for the safeguards can act as brakes on the research schedule—but mistakes, including dangerous ones, are likely to multiply as well.

The headiest increases in research budgets are going into "blue sky" projects not expected to make money for five or ten years. Most of the telecommunications and computer giants have set up semi-autonomous research subsidiaries feeding at the head of the profit stream, and the biotech players are following suit. These spin-offs usually are patterned upon the compartmentalization of the Lockheed "Skunk Works," the top-secret research center that created the F–117 stealth fighter. That way "the left hand knoweth not what the right hand doeth," making it much easier to keep secrets. The river of venture capital pouring into such establishments will be great for surprise product unveilings, but not necessarily for science.

Big Gold Ones

Secrecy works well for another side of business, too. It's a fact of biology that one tenth of all species of plants and animals are parasites. Human parasites are also legion, and the med-tech gold rush will give them marvelous hosts. The secrecy of private industry creates a hospitable climate in which fraud can flourish.

Let's consider the effects of fraud on Medicare costs, which totaled some $212 billion in 1999. Fines and restitution from Columbia/HCA–this is the company that kept double books–are expected to be a tad over a billion. Seven years of double billings from hundreds of hospitals add up to a lot more than that, though. At the company's peak it or its subsidiaries owned almost a tenth of American hospitals, so let's assume that a parasitic tenth ($21 billion) of the Medicare cake had been inflated by 50 percent ("common in the industry") each year for seven years. That's about $50 billion drained directly from taxpayers into the pockets of private health-care criminals. The first-ever decline in Medicare spending in 1999, $20 billion less than predicted, may have been due largely to a temporary chill on fraud emanating from this case.

The hospital conglomerate was not the only double dealer in health care. A 1994 audit of 21 randomly selected hospitals by the Department of Health and Human Services found more than $50 million in Medicare charges unrelated to patient care, including everything from the Thomas Jefferson University Hospital president's rent to "a trip to Italy to inspect a sculpture" for an executive at the Medical College of Pennsylvania. Bulk buys of Christmas gifts were a popular item at every institution.

Extrapolate these findings to the 7,000 hospitals in the United States and you have another $20 billion defrauded from taxpayers each year. And that's *not* counting unwanted medical procedures done on cowed or dying patients strictly for financial reasons. Nor does it include $20 charges for "thermal therapy devices" (ice packs) and the like—the medical equivalents of the Pentagon's $600 toilet seats.

Of necessity, these totals are estimated. Still, they illustrate the kind of money to be made by playing with decimal points in complicated third-party reimbursement systems. And little of it is ever recovered.

In fact, we would like to hear about any fraud settlement or fine that equals or exceeds the amount ripped off, particularly at the upper levels of achievement. The law treats white-collar crime with notorious leniency. Ted C. Fishman, a former currency trader, researched fraud in the financial industry by collecting all those boring little swindles from the news wires and the back pages of the financial press. He found that, on average, one million-dollar fraud comes to light every day, and one $10 million fleece every third day. Securities fraud alone costs American shareholders a million dollars an hour, according to the North American Securities Administrators Association.

At every level of discovery, fraud pays. More is committed than reported. More is reported than traced. And even when fraud is proven, more is stolen than recovered. There's no reason to believe it's any different in the health-care industry.

Indeed, there's plenty of evidence that it's exactly the same. Take "Vitamins Incorporated," the global vitamin scam. Roche Pharmaceuticals (a division of Hoffmann–La Roche), BASF, Rhône-Poulenc, Takeda Chemical Industries, and other makers of bulk vitamins conspired for more than ten years to fix prices, defrauding consumers throughout the world of a sum that can be only vaguely estimated—certainly $5 billion, probably $10 billion, possibly $20 billion. Compared to the profits that the conspiring companies realized, the projected $2 billion in fines and settlements for monopolizing the American market amounts to little more than a speeding ticket.

Roche has been at the game at least since manipulating prices for Valium and Librium in the 1970s. In fact, Roche and its practices are part of a Central European "tradition" of cartel building that goes back to I. G. Farben, the German chemical giant that built a monopoly under the Third Reich.

Roche no doubt will rise from the wrist slapping to fix again. CEO Franz Humer tacitly seemed to promise as much in a truculently opaque statement he made after disclosure of the fraud. He blamed it on a few "rogue executives"—operating in more than a dozen companies through changes of personnel over the course of a decade—then coolly admonished his listeners, "You will understand that this was not part of our responsibility."

And if not the same players, new ones will fill the niche in the business environment. Commodities that are indistinguishable from one company to another as well as vertically integrated industries, in which a few companies control everything from raw material to final product, are especially vulnerable, and few corporate buccaneers can resist the lure of pure profit for so little risk. Molecular medicine will provide them with some 24-karat opportunities, perhaps in the supply of substrates, nutrients, and reagents for biomedical testing and manufacturing.

Nor is pricing the only avenue of profitable deceit being paved with gold in medical heaven. Commercialization has made troubling conflicts of interest endemic in research.

A single doctor often invents a product, designs the clinical trials, presents it at conferences, and touts it in the journals. In the early stages, of course, this may be unavoidable. He's the only one who understands it. And it is legitimately his invention, his property. It's part of his job to convince others of its worth. And if he succeeds in doing so, he thereby draws wealth to the company he partly owns—but only as long as the experimental results are good. That's a powerful incentive to *improve* the results by a little creative manipulation. This temptation is sure to produce some spectacular debacles in the coming decades.

Suppressing unfavorable test results is common in many industries. The recent attempt by Immune Response Corp. of Carlsbad, California, to quash a report showing that its Remune AIDS vaccine doesn't work was a shocker that bodes ill for the future of medicine. After being censured by the FDA in 1995 for fudging a preliminary study, the company hired James Kahn of the University of California at San Francisco and Stephen Lagakos of the Harvard School of Public Health, who conducted the largest AIDS vaccine trial to date from 1996 to 1999. They stopped the test early when it became clear that the vaccine had no effect.

Claiming proprietorship of the facts, Immune Response first demanded that the scientists abandon their report on the failure, then withheld some test tabulations in an effort to prevent publication of the negative findings. Later they tried to get the researchers to include a chart based on invalid statistical methods that showed some benefit. The case is now in arbitration, and the company has asked for $10 million from the scientists as punishment for publishing the facts.

In forming any realistic policy to rein in medical costs, we must budget for fraud, as much as 10 percent in certain sectors. That's not the same as accepting it. The Columbia/HCA case shows it can be made an *intermittent* problem. But by far the hardest challenge for public policymakers as they strive to regulate the new medical science will be keeping the dollars out of the data.

PART TWO

Dangers of Biotech Medicine

CHAPTER 7

Start Saving Now for Your Child's Third Eye!

AS WE'VE ALREADY SUGGESTED, biotechnology will fundamentally change the goals of medicine. After all, to investors, the diseased are just another market. If genetic medicine works well enough to reduce the supply of the solvent sick, it will reduce its own source of profits. To forestall such an outcome, new markets must be opened as quickly as old ones get saturated. And it stands to reason that new technology will be used, by those who can afford it, to give pleasure as well as to take away pain.

Thus, medicine as driven by biotechnology will become more concerned with remodeling, less with repairs. The point when the balance tips in favor of upgrade procedures will come around 2010 or 2015. By then, the geneticist William Hazeltine estimates, well over half of the new medical procedures introduced each year will be elective improvements rather than therapies. Using a few areas of medical research as examples, we'll try to predict some attributes of the new consumer-oriented bionic medicine.

The Genetic Workout

For some years now, doctors have been able to give human growth hormone (HGH) to children deficient in it, in order to prevent dwarfism, abnormally short stature. HGH used to be rare and terribly expensive—it had to be laboriously collected from cadavers—but now it is readily biosynthesized. Dr. Raymond Hintz, a pediatrician who teaches at Stanford University, has shown that it can add height to healthy children who are merely a bit shorter than average. In a 10-year study of 121 children, boys grew two inches taller than predicted from their childhood height and the height of their parents; girls grew two and a half extra inches.

There is no reason tall people can't buy extra inches as well, and genetic manipulation should produce even more dramatic results. Maybe the next generation of basketball players won't even have to jump!

Bionic medicine may make other sports easier, too. Exercise produces specific physiological changes in the body, and there are millions of people who would love to enjoy the benefits of exercise without investing the time and effort. With such huge potential sales, drug makers surely will devise "workout" pills to confer many of the benefits of exercise—better bone density, circulation, metabolic rate, muscle tone, and toxin removal in sweat.

Genetic screening opens up an enormous area of potential improvements in human physiology. The great medical hope behind genetic screening is this: As expertise grows about multigene relationships, doctors may be able not only to predict trouble ahead but also to unravel the biochemical particulars behind an individual's current complaints. A doctor might chart the genetic and psychological variables that have helped make a person fat, for example, then tailor a drug combination to cure the patient's obesity and sidestep today's risky, ineffective diets and pills.

The desperate expectancy of this particular market can be gauged by approval of the fat-blocking drug orlistat, marketed by Hoffmann–La Roche under the trade name Xenical. Though probably of some benefit to some people, this drug would never have made it to market had there been a truly effective alternative.

Orlistat simply doesn't work very well. Weight loss averages just 4 percent, and the pounds come right back if the drug and a low-fat diet are discontinued.

The drug also blocks absorption of fat-soluble vitamins, making supplements essential. It produces nasty side effects, including sudden fecal incontinence, if one should succumb to temptation and eat a fatty meal. It may tend to cause breast cancer. Finally, it costs a lot: $1.10 three times a day for over a year.

That's $1,200 a year, plus the vitamins—plus the other drugs, untested in combination, that many doctors say they'll add to try to get worthwhile results.

Improved weight-loss medications are on the horizon. Researchers recently have found the adipostat, a small group of cells in the hypothalamus that act as a fat-storage thermostat. Mediating between two neuron pathways, one of which stimulates appetite, the other of which inhibits it, the adipostat cells memorize the body's "normal" weight and then tenaciously maintain it.

The problem is that brain cells can't tell the difference between a weight-loss diet and starvation. When "starvation" begins, the adipostat mobilizes all metabolic assets to conserve energy and store every available calorie, trying to get the weight back up. It typically overshoots the mark a bit, which is why most weight-loss diets result in a net gain over time.

Now that we know where the adipostat cells are, drug researchers will be able to direct their efforts more efficiently. One of their early candidates is C75, a drug that was being evaluated for cancer treatment at Johns Hopkins University Medical Center when it showed an unexpected side effect: Test mice lost one fourth of their weight in two or three days. Investigators think C75 may trick the brain into thinking its owner has just eaten.

Customized Flesh

On November 6, 1998, two teams of researchers working independently announced success in growing human embryonic stem cells in the laboratory. This accomplishment opens the way to eventual genetic repair or modification of all human cell types.

Concurrent discoveries about the physical structure of tissues are showing bioengineers how to mimic nature's own manufacturing processes to make new kinds of materials for medical instruments, prostheses, and surgical repair.

Synthetic human skin has been expensively available for burn victims for several years. Researchers have successfully grown cartilage cells on forms made of biodegradable polymers, meaning that soon, artificial implants for damaged ears and noses, or for trick knees and tennis elbows, will be available. Artificial bone, tendon, and ligament have also been made in the lab using a matrix of biodegradable hydrogels (water-absorbent "soggy" proteins) as an injectible, moldable substrate for cells grown in the laboratory. Such a matrix serves as a temporary scaffolding to hold the "starter" or "seed" cells together. Then it gradually disappears as the cells proliferate and establish the normal structure of tissue they compose.

Other scientists have developed "time-release" genes useful in tissue design. Many bacteria use plasmids, rings of DNA, as chemical factories independent of the nucleus. This lets them quickly evolve new enzyme subsystems for changing environments without risk of damage to their basic cellular metabolism.

Researchers are learning how to add customized plasmids to seed cells in a biomatrix. Such cells might, for example, produce a growth hormone that would stimulate them to quickly replace the artificial framework with living flesh. Since code for making the plasmids is not part of the nuclear DNA, the new cells will not have it and output of the hormone will fall off as the original cells die, preventing overgrowth.

Such biomatrices seeded with a patient's own stem cells to avoid immune rejection could reverse bone loss to tighten or reattach teeth and hasten the notoriously slow healing of ligament and tendon injuries. They would aid in surgical repair of injuries and might outdo electrostimulation in knitting recalcitrant broken bones.

Computer-designed, laser-sculpted implants of metallic and ceramic foams will follow as substrates for entire bones in prosthetic limbs of the future. Already, tissue engineers are visualizing a steady march of technique to true off-the-shelf organs. A group of scientists under Michael V. Sefton of the University of Toronto is planning the research needed to grow hearts, conceived as a ten- to twenty-year project.

One of the biggest problems is how to create a blood supply for artificial organs. A solution is near. Joseph Vacanti and his partners at Boston's Massachusetts General Hospital and the Center for Innovative Minimally Invasive Therapy have etched circulatory channels on silicon chips, then seeded them with cells to grow arteries, veins, and capillaries. Arrays of such chips, no doubt soon to be replaced by gradually dissolving polymer matrices, will be used to grow circulatory systems in experimental organs.

In time, bioengineers will grow tissues and organs with unprecedented capabilities, beginning soon with live-cell implants to secrete a constant supply of a drug. This technique is made possible by the development of small, implantable capsules that hold living cells. The capsules are made of hyperthin plastic film, which acts like a semipermeable membrane. Suppose a group of cells that produce endorphins is surrounded by such a "smart" capsule. The film's selective membrane qualities can shield these cells from the patient's immune system while they deliver the endorphins—or any desired molecules, natural or synthetic—continuously to any part of the body where they're needed, without sending them through the bloodstream to where they're not. This technique is launching a whole new branch of pharmacotherapeutics, one that is expected to produce a quantum leap in the power and safety of *all* drug therapies during the first decade of the twenty-first century.

At present, researchers are testing several cell-capsule models on humans; one is designed to deliver pain relief; another, to treat certain liver diseases. In the near future, encapsulated insulin-producing cells will treat childhood-onset diabetes. Implants of other cells will restore neurotransmitters lost in degenerative nerve diseases like parkinsonism and Huntington's chorea (progressive and fatal dementia). They also may replace visual pigment–producing cells lost in atrophy of the macula lutea, or "yellow spot," the sensitive focal area of the retina whose degeneration is a leading cause of blindness.

Eventually cell capsules will deliver round-the-clock psychiatric drugs so patients can't forget them or avoid taking them by hiding pills under their tongues. The technology may well bring the issue of involuntary treatment of prisoners and the mentally ill to the forefront again.

Other cells will be modified and cultured in vats to serve as factories for all our enzymes and hormones. Still others will be redesigned as living interfaces to sensors and computers, or as extensions of our own native senses. For example, enhanced retinal cells may enable us to see ultraviolet and infrared light waves, as do birds and bees. Redesigned cochleal cells might be implanted as radio, TV, and Internet receivers. They could even be branded, preset to receive a given network's frequencies. Are you old enough to remember the "X-ray specs" sold on the back cover of comic books? Your grandchildren's comics might be hawking X-ray eyes.

Many organisms, from certain bacteria up to birds and people, possess an organ that orients its owner with the earth's magnetic field. In humans it seems to serve as an unconscious direction finder that supplements spatial memory, visual cues, and sun position. New neural connectors might enable us to feel magnetism consciously. Development of vestigial or emergent senses—psychic abilities among them?—is one of the most fascinating projects that researchers in genetic medicine might contemplate.

Medicine Imitates Life

Tissue engineering can be considered part of a larger field called *biomimetics* ("life imitation"), a branch of biotechnology that blurs the distinction between living and nonliving. For a glimpse of the way it will revolutionize production of medical and nonmedical materials, consider the Canadian geneticist Jeffrey Turner's goats.

Turner has implanted genes for making spider silk—for its weight the strongest material on earth—in goat mammary glands. The silk, skimmed from the milk in quantities unobtainable from spiders, will have many uses: surgical sutures, prosthetic bone and tendon, structural matrix for artificial organs, fishing line, cables many times stronger than steel or nylon, industrial safety nets, bulletproof vests, ultralight building materials for airplanes and gossamer architecture, perhaps nets flung into the stratosphere to catch incoming missiles, even runless pantyhose. It is being marketed under the trade name BioSteel by Turner's company, Nexia Biotechnologies of Quebec.

In like manner, the paradigm in most industries will shift from making products to growing them. The line between medical and consumer products will get fuzzy as we go from artificially grown breast prostheses to autonomous milk-producing mammaries to kitchen-counter cows; from hospital rooms that are semiliving 24/7 nurse's assistants to homes that are smarter than we are and cars that incorporate a chauffeur who does the grocery shopping. Materials that possess some attributes of life (like self-replication) without others (like self-direction) will manufacture themselves.

Biomimetics will give rise to entirely new kinds of medical devices. One will regulate the flow of gastric acid for ulcer patients by stimulating or quieting the vagus nerve. Combined with cell capsules, another will deliver metered drips of a drug in response to its concentration in the bloodstream. Cardiac pacemakers will improve, and tiny pumps will relieve pressure from blocked flow of venous blood or cerebrospinal fluid.

Current silicon chip–making technology is likely to reach its limit around 2010. But by then, biomimetics will let chip designers build their circuits from one-molecule-thick films and strands of conductor metals, making it possible to pack thousands of times as many components into the same space. The power and small size of these chips will open up new medical uses for computers implanted in the body—for example, to manage an internal treatment regimen of many interacting drugs and genes, its program wirelessly updatable in the doctor's office.

Molecular films are an example of *nanotechnology*, the new craft of building ultrasmall machines. Already there are computerized microtweezers that can put a gear on an axle inside a tube thinner than a human hair. Tiny bags the size of bacteria have been developed as microscopic test tubes. These vesicles let scientists study chemical reactions as they occur when confined within a living cell; they often proceed differently when they occur within a large volume, such as the bloodstream.

135

These are forerunners of a new industry of micro-electrical-mechanical systems (MEMS). In the 2010s, doctors will be using computerized robots smaller than red blood cells. They'll be sold in pipettes of saline, programmed to perform certain diagnostic tests when injected. They might read out the data when extracted in a blood sample taken later, or they might transmit it continuously by radio to a sensor outside the patient's body.

Tomorrow's nanotechnologists will build complex micromachines by directly manipulating molecules as if they were Tinker Toys. The resultant nanobots would be like dedicated mechanical bacteria. One type might be programmed to scour away arteriosclerotic plaque. Some would chew up blood clots, kidney stones, gallstones, and dental plaque. Others would repair broken capillaries, move fat globules from adipose tissue to the feces, or fight fatigue by helping muscle cells get rid of lactic acid. Still others might work on the outside of the body. Cosmetic nanobots spread over the body in a lotion might give you a constant, automatic shower by cleaning oil and dirt from your skin. One strain might keep the hair on your head trimmed to a chosen length while another kept your chin or legs shaved always smooth as an egg.

Life Extension

Longevity medicine is both the ultimate therapy and the ultimate upgrade. In theory, complete annotated gene maps and supplies of stem cells eventually could enable physicians to repair all tissues and organs as they wear out, thereby extending life span indefinitely while preventing the decrepitude of aging all the way to the end.

"Indefinitely" in this context really means "up to some prepro-grammed limit that is not yet understood." The natural life spans of most multicellular animals, including the human being's three-score and ten, amount to roughly the same number of heart-beats–about 2 or 3 billion, although a few species vary considerably from that total. In general, slower-beating hearts seem to last longer than fast-beating ones.

Many have studied the effects of various factors on longevity. In the late sixties, a gerontologist, Roy Walford, found that mice live 40 percent longer on a diet of 30 percent fewer calories than normal. Others have shown that much of the deterioration of ag-ing is caused by free radicals, highly reactive by-products of me-tabolism, especially of fats. Free radicals cause oxygen damage to cell structures, including DNA. (Think of them as burning ciga-rette holes in your genes.) Thus, the decline of aging can be slowed by free radical-dousing nutrients like vitamin E, vitamin C, beta carotene, and lycopene, or by hibernation, a low-fat diet, or the greater metabolic efficiency and slower pulse that result from regular exercise.

Now genomic science is showing us *how* curtailing free radi-cals slows aging. Early in 2000, the biochemist Leonard Guarente and his coworkers at the Massachusetts Institute of Technology found that nicotinamide adenine dinucleotide (NAD), an impor-tant part of the cell chemistry that burns glucose for energy, also teams up with a protein called sir2 (silent information regulator number 2). With the aid of chromatin, a color-stainable packing material that encloses and protects each chromosome, they let the cell open up or seal off long stretches of DNA. The sir2–NAD duo adds or removes molecular fragments that act as spacers be-tween the DNA and the chromatin, thus allowing or blocking ac-cess to the genes by the transcription enzymes that turn genetic instructions into proteins. By raising NAD levels, a low-calorie diet may close off whole suites of genes used in metabolism, in effect making some cells hibernate to conserve energy and limit free-radical output.

Later that same year Gary Ruvkin and his colleagues at Harvard Medical School found an appetite-related brain hormone in roundworms that shuts off a gene that maintains insulin receptors on cell membranes. As the worm gets hungry, levels of the hormone increase, and the worm burns less glucose. As a result, it makes fewer free radicals and lives longer to ride out famine until it can get enough food to activate its reproductive system.

However, we won't be able to stop aging entirely by eliminating free radicals. Throwing some cold water on the hope for simple solutions, the immune system uses free radicals to kill bacteria, so having too few of them raises the risk of death from infection.

A great deal of life-extension research focuses on the phenomenon of *apoptosis,* the normal death of cells for replacement by new ones in a process of continuous renewal. Apoptosis seems to be controlled by a group of "death genes," activated by the telomeres, identical DNA sequences, a succession of which caps each end of a chromosome like the aglets on the ends of shoelaces. Every cell division knocks off a few of the telomeres, and the theory is that when they're all gone, the death genes kill the cell.

Most researchers think it's the telomeres that restrict differentiated cells to their apparently fixed allotment of 50 divisions (the Hayflick limit), accelerating the body's decline after the reproductive years and eventually shutting down vital functions altogether. Timed hormonal signals from the brain may regulate the speed of the process, and various chemical pathways probably expedite or inhibit it. Natural selection created the death system, evolutionary biologists believe, to deal with sex—that is, to make the length of reproductive cycles fit various ecological niches, and to make room and board available for each new generation by clearing away the old.

Of course, if eternal life means fasting and celibacy, death begins to look a lot more attractive. However, there may be some loopholes in our genetic lease on life. Future drugs may be made to dampen the sir2-NAD system, or the hormone in the cell membrane that silences the insulin-receptor gene, or some other chemical pathway, without decreasing energy levels too much.

In December 2000, researchers under Stephen L. Helfand of the University of Connecticut Health Center in Farmington reported a lead to such a chemical pathway from work with fruit flies. The researchers accidentally mutated a gene for a protein that carries nutrients through the cell membrane into the interior of cells. The mutation slightly lowered the efficiency of the transport protein, in effect lowering food intake without restricting the flies' diet. The change nearly doubled the insects' average life span and raised their maximum life span by 50 percent. The gene, which Helfand's group called INDY, for I'm Not Dead Yet, exists in humans and could be an eventual target for a longevity drug.

In November 1999, a team under Pier Giuseppe Pelicci of the European Institute of Oncology in Milan announced the discovery of one of the death genes, a stretch of DNA in mice that makes a protein that starts apoptosis when the mouse's genetic proofreader finds free-radical damage. When Pelicci turned off the gene, the mice lived 30 percent longer. This gene's protein belongs to a class of cellular trigger proteins already well studied, so pharmacologists will have a head start in devising a life-extension drug to block it.

Some of the most hopeful leads come from cloning research.

When researchers at Edinburgh's Roslin Institute cloned a sheep, the clone, Dolly, had fewer telomeres than the ewe she was cloned from. But Robert Lanza and Michael West of Advanced Cell Technologies in Worcester, Massachusetts, reported in April 2000 that six cloned cows did *not* show the reduced number of telomeres found in Dolly. Quite the contrary, the calves had 50 percent *more* telomeres than normal. No one knows why yet. On the basis of the extra number of telomeres it can be estimated that these animals might live to about 35, the human equivalent of 120 years.

From embryonic stem cells, several biologists have extracted telomerase, the enzyme that restores the telomeres and enables stem cells to divide without limit. It's now known that some mammalian cells cycle continuously from embryonic cells to germ (sperm and egg) cells and back again, and so, like some of the most primitive amoebas, they never die of natural causes.

Thus there may be many routes to life-prolonging drugs. One day it may even be possible to reset the human aging clock, causing the entire body to rejuvenate itself indefinitely. Medicine would then have realized its ultimate goal: a vaccine against death.

Side Effects of Success?

Commercial medicine has embarked on a truly awesome endeavor. As we surveyed the estimated two thousand companies and the even larger number of universities and government centers currently doing medical research, we were reminded of one of those striking photos of the pit mines of the Brazilian gold rush during the 1980s. At first glance, the picture looks like a large hole in the ground completely covered with thousands of ants. Then something clicks, you get a sense of the true scale, and you realize that it's a *vast* hole and each ant is a man, working with hammer, shovel, and sieve at his own tiny piece of the dream.

Medical treasure is being unearthed in the biotechnology gold rush, but there may be long-term social side effects.

Suppose genetic medicine is more successful than even its most ardent proponents hope. Let's say it proceeds smoothly from triumph to triumph. Doctors can cure previously incurable diseases, make people immune to the effects of eating saturated fats, increase their strength, and double their IQs, without side effects or gene spills along the way. Let's further suppose that, as with computers, new methods yield unforeseen economies, and "gene pills" become as cheap as vitamins.

Won't readily available upgrades drain some of the specialness out of talent and beauty? Or simply raise the bar? What will be the cumulative effect on the human race if the solutions to life's problems become easy? Would it still mean anything to pursue meditation, academic study, athletic training, or piano practice? Do we then lose some essential drive? Are there genes for will and perseverance?

The "new retail" approach to medicine discussed in Chapter 3 will apply most to genetic-upgrade. Some parents will second-mortgage the house to give their children better genes, as they do now to pay for tuition to top universities. Will cognitive "finishing" become a prerequisite for admission to the best colleges? Perhaps schools and sports teams will try to even the odds a little with "gene scholarships" for those who show exceptional promise even while unmodified.

Many genetic upgrades will confer a great competitive advantage on those who can pay for them. Does this mean that wealth will confer even greater advantages than heretofore? What becomes of America's cherished Horatio Alger image? Are we thus to become a nation, a world, of genetic underdogs and *Übermenschen*?

A further point to consider is that genetic medicine eventually will treat the unborn as well as the born. Will this risk splitting upper from lower class even further, perhaps to the extent that eventually they will become two species, like the leisured Eloi and subterranean Morlock toilers of H. G. Wells's classic novella, *The Time Machine*? Bypassing natural selection, germ-cell modification combined with the accelerated selection of the marketplace might accomplish such a thing in a century or two.

What effect would longevity treatments have in such a world? Organ transplants, stem-cell injections, and whole-body enzyme-restoration treatments will be among molecular medicine's most expensive procedures. The rich only used to get richer. Soon they'll be getting taller and smarter, and then they'll live longer.

An immortal minority would be one more demographic pressure on medical costs, but that's the least of it. Death always has been the great democratizer. What now, if money equals life? In 1984, the governor of Colorado, Richard Lamm, raised a storm of controversy when he said the elderly and terminally ill have "a duty to die and get out of the way." In the future that duty may be shared by the terminally poor. As time becomes the ultimate medical commodity, will it be offered on a "pay as you stay" basis? If you lose your money in a stock market crash, will your doctor push you out the window?

CHAPTER 8

Personal Alchemy

BIOTECHNOLOGY IS CREATING HUGE new arenas of medical commerce. Much of this commerce will consist of what we have termed "upgrade medicine" to distinguish it from therapeutic medicine: upgrade medicine is treatments designed to alleviate feelings of dissatisfaction about one's body, emotions, or intellectual abilities. The medicine of the future promises a kind of alchemy, magically transmuting the "lead" of a person's present characteristics into the "gold" of traits he or she wishes to possess.

For an advance glimpse of the social side effects of this upgrade medicine, the recent history of cosmetic surgery is informative.

Since 1992, the size of this field, as measured in dollars and number of operations, has at least doubled. The true increase may be much greater, since current statistics are collected only from plastic surgeons, not from other doctors who also do cosmetic work. The most common procedures, liposuction and breast reconfiguration, are now performed three times as often as they were at the beginning of the decade, and often on younger patients.

The explosion is due in part to the fact that cosmetic surgeons have become savvy marketers. For one thing, they are working hard to make men a larger part of their patient base, trading on masculine bodily insecurities that are expertly addressed in four-color brochures featuring Aphrodite on the arm of This-Could-Be-You. As of 1997, men's spending on the most popular unisex procedures–face-lifts and liposuction–had risen to 15 percent of women's, with further growth on the horizon.

Even dubious male-only procedures are finding a marketplace. Despite high risk of deformity, excruciating pain, and poor results even in the best of cases, American men are spending at least $20 million a year on penile-enlargement surgery. Imagine the extent of the market for an equivalent technique that really works.

Elective operations such as plastic surgery are not regulated the way medically necessary surgery is. Any M.D. can buy some equipment on credit, hang out a shingle on the Web or in the Yellow Pages, and become a plastic surgeon. There's no need for hospital affiliation, with its peer-review panels, and most states don't require certification by the American Board of Medical Specialties or other professional groups.

The doctor may do no more than take a weekend seminar given by the equipment maker and still be legally qualified in most states to do liposuction, laser surgery, and all the rest. Finance companies specializing in medical loans put "Why wait?" banners on the doctor's Web page. In this free-for-all market, 1 of every 5,000 liposuction clients dies, 10 percent of all cosmetic procedures must be redone, and the best plastic surgeons spend one fifth of their time trying to salvage the handiwork of their incompetent colleagues.

The demand for plastic surgery is often so emotionally urgent that many show less caution shopping for a face-lift than for a fax machine. The self-improvement medicine of the future, fueled by the techniques and discoveries of genomic science, will have the same emotional appeal, with higher profits to providers and more hype and marketing muscle behind it.

Desire Versus Need

In medicine, it is becoming ever harder to disentangle desire from need. The very meaning of the words often seems to differ by economic status. In the upper-middle class, the trend is to consider cosmetic surgery a kind of necessity, an ongoing maintenance project like the annual physical—a touch-up to go with the checkup. To those in the lower economic echelons, it often feels more like the purchase of a heavily mortgaged house in a neighborhood that's a little *too* expensive—a much-desired symbol of upward mobility that produces a long struggle between keeping up appearances and keeping up the payments.

The waters get further muddied by crossover, the phenomenon by which treatments developed in response to a medical need often find a much larger market based on desire; an example is the use of human growth hormone to enhance healthy physiques instead of to correct major mistakes of Mother Nature. The readiness to make this shift is probably a natural human trait, augmented by advertising and by social forces like the Baby Boomers' entitlement syndrome, discussed in Chapter 2. Today steroids are used far more by bodybuilders than by their originally intended users, patients fighting wasting illnesses. If Viagra had been prescribed only for clinically assessed erectile dysfunction and not for extra added assurance, hardness, and durability, it never would've become such a success.

The crossover of need into desire often leads us to ask more of drugs than they can accomplish. Though it was the first superstar of the new personal alchemy, Viagra is no cure-all for sexual problems. Nor can Viagra generate attraction between two specific people, as did the potions of popular song and ancient legend, no matter how much the pair might want it to. Indeed, the drug's erectile effectiveness for most of its users can lead to devastating disappointment for those couples whom it fails to help.

Overreliance on drugs also tempts us to neglect causative factors. Viagra's quick-fix power can lead people to disregard emotional problems or the lack of free time and so miss the source of their difficulty, as well as bypassing a chance for greater closeness. In this respect it teaches us to expect some recoil from medicine's magic bullets.

When a new medical treatment solves a problem, we get excited. Seldom do we think about its potential to create new problems with injudicious use, yet the possibility is almost always there. It's the downside of crossover, which we might call the backfire effect.

We have a perfect example of the backfire effect in the waning effectiveness of antibiotics. Patients' demand, and doctors' inability to resist it, has led to a four-decade binge of overprescription, as well as the mass dosing with antibiotics of animals used for meat. Owing to their magical reputation, hijacked shipments of the drugs often are hawked along Third World roadsides as cures for everything from alopecia to zymosis.

Children often get the worst of it. Physicians want parents to see that they are "doing something," even though the doctors know that antibiotics affect only bacteria, not the viruses that cause most of children's ailments, like colds and flu. As a result, bacteria have rapidly evolved resistance to antibiotics, and some of those most dangerous to the young and the elderly, like *Streptococcus pneumoniae* and *Staphylococcus* species, are leading the way.

Perhaps the most common example of crossover is the use of drugs for their psychological effects. In the culture of the Native Americans of the Southwest, peyote was used as both medicine and vision inducer. In our own culture, opiates once were used to give relief to pain, and a larger number took, and take, the same drugs (at least initially) for pleasure. When life is hard, the absence of pain *is* pleasure, so the terms are bound to blur.

In the world of psychoactive drugs, crossover affects all classes and social groups, with huge economic, political, and legal consequences, many of them malign. Consensus about how to regard these molecules that magically change our moods may forever elude us, yet it's clear that when we push the desire for mood-altering substances into the shadows through prohibition, we make the drugs much more expensive, which generates greater profits for smugglers, ropes enforcers and smugglers into a deadly war dance, and exacts a terrible price in money and lives. Meanwhile, the medical benefits of the drugs themselves are lost.

A similar thicket of ethical and social problems arises when the desire for a medical procedure or treatment results from irrational fears or when it involves problems that might better be avoided than treated. The speed and power of tomorrow's new medical fixes will inevitably increase our fondness for the easy way out, which often proves in the long run to be the hard way.

Freedom from Fear?

Consider this quick-fix dynamic in the mania for prescribing methylphenidate (sold as Ritalin, among other brand names), fluoxetine (Prozac), and other drugs used for treating hyperactivity and attention deficit disorder (ADD). First they were given to teenagers, then to elementary-school pupils, and now they are routinely prescribed for preschoolers. The trend to administer powerful drugs to an ever younger population is so pronounced as to provoke dismay from the American Medical Association, the White House, parents, teachers—and even some crocodile tears from the manufacturers.

Childhood learning difficulties are blamed variously on genetics, food additives, sugar, caffeine (almost ubiquitous in soft drinks), urban stress, boring schools, and our jump-cut video world, with good evidence for contributions by all of the above. Some suggest that children are suffering from loss of childhood, feeling coerced into preparing for college from the age of four instead of just being allowed to play.

Perhaps redesigning the environment in which we raise our

offspring is worth considering. But few people talk about this, and fewer still try to act on it.

The discovery and marketing of ADD as a "disorder" raises more general questions: To what extent do we want medicine to be a substitute for self-discipline, healthy living, and a caring society? How should we choose which "medical" needs to service medically and which to treat through old-fashioned nonmedical means?

Some related questions: How will behavior be affected by the increasing availability of medical treatments for supposed behavioral ills? Will we drink more when we know that alcoholism and cirrhosis can be cured? Will a vaccine against tooth decay lead to an increase in sugar consumption? Would the advent of a truly effective weight-control drug usher in a bull market for companies that make ice cream and candy? Do we want our lives to be better, or just better medicated?

These questions suggest the need for an across-the-board examination of the market for psychiatric drugs. Anxiety and depression, the most common mental illnesses among the U.S. population, are examples of problems that our system treats only downstream, at the individual level, instead of striving to prevent them upstream, at the social level.

Brain researchers have found that traumatic events in childhood are encoded into synaptic patterns in the amygdala, the brain's fear center. There they lodge, hidden from consciousness, causing the adult a vertiginous array of phobias, anxieties, and dysfunctions.

Many of those who study rape and incest estimate that one fifth to one third of girls and one seventh to one fourth of boys in the United States have been sexually molested by the end of adolescence. The experience often has devastating effects on their ability to form intimate relationships as adults. Many other children are spanked, slapped, or beaten without overt sexual trauma. Later they have twice the average rate of alcoholism, drug addiction, and anxiety disorders. Brutality toward children is also a major cause of obesity and sexual dysfunction.

In the century since Freud, psychology has made great strides in elucidating the effects of such abuse. Yet psychotherapy has failed to find a reliable way to undo the damage. And recent discoveries about the genetic components of anxiety and depression, along with the success of Prozac and its cousins, which work for about 60 percent of patients, have led many to discard all cognitive approaches as worthless. The willingness of some therapists to treat patients for years without visible results has left a black mark on their profession. One patient who found that she felt better when she was prescribed Prozac even sued her shrink for wasting her time and money on the "talking cure." Yet the continuing widespread abuse of children is likely to limit the long-term effectiveness of chemical treatment of the results.

Pharmacologists soon will create drugs to erase deep-seated irrational fears left over from the past. Will they also delete parts of the fear response itself—what we might term our rational fears? After all, a proper dose of fear at the right time can save your life from a charging rhino or a glittery-eyed sociopath.

Fear plays an important part in public awareness, too. Even the much-derided "conspiracy buffs" sometimes turn out to be right. Mind adjusters that affect the fear circuits would be perfectly adapted to perform a hidden function: erasure of suspicion and skepticism among the multitudes, giving our rulers a freer hand.

Judiciously used, selective fear-deletion drugs could be a marvelous tool that would benefit millions. Given our tendency to worship the quick fix, however, they may have insidious dangers, keeping us from dealing with root causes of our individual, social, and political ills. Of course, *that* would raise and perpetuate the demand for more drugs.

A specific kind of fear—social phobia, a debilitating shyness so extreme as to prevent nearly all interaction with other people—afflicts at least 12 million Americans permanently, and an estimated 35 million at some point in their lives. It typically begins with humiliating teenage social catastrophes, setting the pattern for adult loneliness. Use of popular antidepressants to treat it has given those drugs a second wind in the sales marathon.

Demand for mood-altering drugs can only grow, given the fact that our society is evolving in ways that seem guaranteed to produce higher levels of loneliness, alienation, and social anxiety. For the foreseeable future, one of everyone's key struggles will be against those who seek to frustrate human needs by playing on our fears, then medicalize the resulting frustrations into profitable disorders.

Dosing Away the Sadness

Many new "outlook drugs," drugs that go beyond the mood alterants of the past, will be released in the next decade. Psychiatrists hope that these drugs will make it possible to reshape personality by changing the balance among the brain's neurotransmitters, making patients more assertive, serene, optimistic, and so on, all faster and more effectively than is possible through arduous psychotherapy or yogic mental training.

This drug bonanza will include a wider range of treatments for depression. Many sufferers have not been helped by the last big advance, the serotonin reuptake inhibitors (SRIs) such as Prozac, Zoloft, Luvox, and Paxil. Others love the results at first but later find they've entered an emotional twilight zone where they are indeed no longer sad because they can't feel much of anything at all and nothing matters much one way or another. Since one in eight Americans is depressed, this market alone starts at 35 million potential customers.

New drugs may benefit many of the 40 percent of depressives for whom current drugs fail. Nevertheless, the best psychiatrists readily admit that we still know far too little about neurotransmitters to make treatment of depression an exact science anytime soon.

Once again, we'll need to balance spectacular benefits for some against possible damage to others and against the general dangers of overuse and misuse. We must remember that psychiatric drugs have helped many people get their bearings in life, some of whom have eloquently described their gratitude to the pharmaceutical companies. One such person is Kelly Luker, a journalist who contributed the following testimony in an essay for *Salon.com*:

> One or two Prozac a day is the chemical equivalent of my beloved chenille throw and a hot cup of soup on a rainy day. It is the sense of comfort replacing almost a lifetime of dread. And glory be, my brain works again. I can now read a menu without bursting into tears over the pressure of having to make a decision.

We must try to minimize abuse without curtailing availability to those in crisis. Still, like the spreading use of antianxiety drugs to treat fears and worries once considered aspects of the human condition, the medicalization of depression also has troubling implications for social control.

Scientists are gradually uncovering genetic predispositions to depression, which will probably be amenable to biochemical modification one day soon. Genes, it may be said, are the master, the composer who sets out the orchestration for our internal music. Yet genes are also the servants, the musicians who play the neurotransmitter symphony according to the score of our thoughts and experiences. It's a complex mutualism that words can't capture. Consider this conundrum: Impotence, lack of desire, and inability to reach orgasm are recognized as both causes and effects of depression. Yet many patients who use SRIs develop these symptoms as side effects. We'll make some colossal blunders if we use our new genomic knowledge to interfere in this system hastily or carelessly, mistaking the metaphor for the music.

Like fear, depression is sometimes more a danger signal than a disease. It may mean that one's creativity is being stifled, and one needs to change one's way of life. Very few in our malled and cubicled world can stay thoroughly grounded in the sensory stimuli of their native planet. Even fewer get a chance to do work they love. The statistically most significant contributor to physical and mental health—fulfilling intimacy with a lover—turns out to be a mirage for most people.

One person in eight is depressed? A philosopher might wonder why the ratio is so low. Perhaps a rush to obliterate the problem medically isn't the path our society should be heading down.

CHAPTER 9

Living Commodities

LOOKING INTO THE FUTURE OF GE-
netic medicine, many people are
alarmed by the prospect of designer babies–children assembled from a menu
of traits and aptitudes like pizzas with
selected toppings. Collectively we're trying to decide whether there's anything
intrinsically wrong with the idea or
whether it's merely strange and new.

Two decades ago, according to opinion polls, in vitro fertilization seemed

horrifyingly unnatural to most people. Today it's just another way to start a life, and a great blessing to the otherwise childless. Now the recently developed ability to grow transplanted human eggs in mice seems less outlandish than it once would have. The technique enables women likely to be rendered infertile by cancer treatment or endometriosis to preserve their own eggs and so have children that carry their mother's genes. Offspring design may follow the same curve of acceptance.

Most of the objections center on two fears—that of turning personality into merchandise and that of "playing God."

In the context of consumer capitalism, it would be hard to think of any aspect of personality that is not already commercialized to some degree. Moreover, most parents try to equip their children with the traits needed to prosper in a competitive world. Genetic planning seems like a logical extension of the motives and methods by which people already shape their progeny. Is creating a child as a work of art any worse than making one as an heir or as a surrogate fulfiller of one's own abandoned dreams?

The fear of becoming "as gods" crops up with almost every new technology. "If God had meant us to fly, He would have given us wings." Well, She did give us minds, so perhaps we were meant to soar after all. Few people today consider heavier-than-air flight a sign of hubris.

A portion of the "as gods" fear is quite rational. It's a dread of making fateful mistakes, perhaps *worse* mistakes than those made by nature. It's the collective feeling of being unready or out of control, possibilities that are hard to dismiss.

However, part of that argument seems to be simple fear of success, a feeling that it's not right to dodge our share of misfortune. The usual cure for that problem is a larger dose of success.

Today's science already contains hints of the triumphs of reproductive planning in the decades to come. Consider, for example, the technique of preimplantation genetic diagnosis (PGD), available since 1999.

Aneuploidy (extra copies of chromosomes) and transposition (lengths of DNA switched between chromosomes) are the leading causes of stillbirths, especially in older women. PGD has made great strides in weeding out embryos with these faults and thus enabling older women to bear healthy babies. In September 2000, PGD made it possible for one child to save the life of another when a transplant of umbilical cord cells from a newborn infant, Adam Nash, cured his seven-year-old sister, Molly, of Fanconi's anemia, a fatal lack in the bone marrow of progenitor cells for red blood cells.

We may rightly worry that the technique will be abused in the future, inducing people to make babies only as sources of spare parts for siblings, perhaps leading to reservoirs of girls in lands where only boys are valued. (Unlikely, you say? The poor already sell kidneys to the rich, and testicle transplants are just around the corner.) But for now let us glory in a medical wonder that gave one doomed child the chance for a full life.

Gender Selection

It is much less clear how genetic design will change society. Once it becomes a matter of choice, will we stock the gene pool with an interesting mix or will it be all angelfish and sharks? Many traits exist as a gradient between two poles of excess: a healthy spirit of adventure flanked by recklessness and timidity, for example; industry between mania and torpor. Will the vogue for equivocal traits rise and fall like hemlines?

Countries with national health plans will be able to sculpt the genetic market from above by prohibiting certain procedures and adjusting the entrance requirements for others. In countries where ideology favors the unfettered operation of the market-place, financial factors will play a leading role. Two Israeli fertil-ity-clinic doctors were recently arrested for harvesting extra eggs for resale without their clients' knowledge. In the land of free en-terprise, prime germ cells might someday be listed on the com-modities market alongside pork bellies. Bidding for supermodel eggs and college-football-player sperm already has begun at $50,000 per unit.

Our very limited early experience with child design offers little on which to base a forecast. In a 1998 survey by the New En-gland Regional Genetics Group, only 11 percent of parents said they would abort a fetus having a genetic predisposition to obe-sity. Of course, the percentage might be much higher if the abor-tion could be by means of a noninvasive method just after conception.

Microsort, a technique that lets couples determine the sex of a baby-to-be with 80 to 90 percent accuracy, has been available for a couple of years. Developed first for cattle breeding, it involves staining the DNA in a sperm sample with a fluorescent dye, then using a laser-driven machine to sort, one by one, the "male" sperm cells–those carrying the Y chromosome–from the "fe-males." (Because the Y chromosome is smaller than the X, sperm cells carrying the Y chromosome have slightly less DNA and therefore glow a bit less brightly.)

So far, demand for boys and girls has been about equal. How-ever, that may be because the sole practitioner licensed to use the technique, the Genetics and IVF Institute of Fairfax, Virginia, accepts only clients who wish to balance the number of boys and girls in their families.

At about $7,500 per conception, Microsort is not likely to affect society's gender ratio anytime soon. But when 100 percent accurate sex determination is readily available for a tenth of that price, as it likely will be by 2005, the social effects may be significant. In India and China, amniocentesis (analysis of the amniotic fluid) and abortion are so widely used to prevent the birth of girls that bride prices are rising rapidly. In the United States, a majority of families believe that a male firstborn is the ideal. Primacy in birth order confers numerous advantages on the firstborn, including a tendency toward the aggressive dominance so valued in our culture. Thus, gender selection via genetic planning could lead to more aggressive firstborn males, which would worsen some of the problems that women have struggled so hard to overcome.

Germ-Line Therapy

Certain hereditary diseases are sex-linked, that is, determined by genes on the X or Y chromosome, so gender selection can sometimes be used as preventive medicine. In fact, this has already been done by doctors in Barcelona who enabled a hemophiliac to be sure of fathering a son—triplets, as it turned out—so as to avoid the danger of passing on the disease to future generations by fathering a daughter. This way, the sons cannot inherit hemophilia and cannot bequeath the gene to their children. Females do not suffer from hemophilia, but they can pass the gene on to their male offspring.

Hemophilia is caused by a recessive defect on the X chromosome. The disease itself normally appears only in men, when a son inherits a flawed X chromosome from his mother. A woman with one defective X chromosome is a carrier of the malady, but in her the presence of another, intact, X chromosome prevents the blood-clotting problem from manifesting itself in her body.

In this case, the researchers took a single cell from each of three early in vitro embryos and checked it to make sure it carried a Y (male) chromosome. Against the odds, all three embryos were male, and all three were successfully implanted in the mother's womb and carried to term. Soon gender selection will routinely let mutation carriers avoid having children who manifest or carry other sex-linked diseases like hydrocephalus, Duchenne's muscular dystrophy, and fragile-X syndrome.

Testing of embryos for these and other inherited conditions is now becoming available, and such therapeutic purposes will drive the genetic-planning industry in its early years. The next logical step is to introduce modified genes into germ cells or young embryos, thereby preventing diseases before they arise. This process is called germ-line therapy.

Several laboratories are developing artificial wombs, which would open the door to motherhood for millions of woman whose reproductive organs have been damaged by genetic defect, disease, or injury. Such a controlled environment also will be ideal for studying experimental fetuses. Embryologists will use womb pods to study the effect of germ-cell genetic changes in animals and, when possible, humans.

Germ-cell modification may turn out to be the best way to do genetic therapy. It would be necessary to change genes in only one or two cells, instead of using vectors to change billions of cells in a whole organ. The methods will be tried out and perfected first in animals. Chromos Molecular Systems of Burnaby, British Columbia, is one of several companies developing germ-line procedures to create genetically modified cows and goats capable of producing drugs and human hormones in their milk or blood.

Already, however, the era of human germ-line therapy has begun. At least 30 babies have been born with modified DNA–but in the mitochondria, the cells' energy plants, rather than the germ-cell nuclei. The procedure, developed at the Institute for Reproductive Medicine and Science of Saint Barnabas, in West Orange, New Jersey, corrects a defect in maternal mitochondrial DNA that causes infertility. No ill effects have been noted from the treatment.

Laymen and scientists alike are wary of germ-line therapy owing to its potential for side effects in future generations. Mario Capecchi of the University of Utah has devised a prototype process designed to sidestep that danger. He flanks a therapeutic gene with "scissor genes," activated by enzymes produced only in developing sperm and eggs. Thus, a genetic change could be introduced into a fertilized egg or early embryo and do its work throughout a person's life, then be automatically deleted from that individual's reproductive cells at maturity.

However, other pitfalls may appear. One method of fertilization that would be used in germ-line therapy is intracytoplasmic sperm injection (ICSI, pronounced "ICK-see"), which is already used to overcome about 20,000 cases of male infertility every year in the United States. Normally, a motile sperm extrudes its nucleus into an egg, leaving the DNA's cellular coat and tail at the door. In ICSI, doctors squirt a whole sperm cell into the egg. The problem is that viruses can stick tenaciously to the outside of the sperm and may be introduced into the fertilized egg, either killing the embryo or dooming the new individual to any of various viral diseases, including AIDS and certain cancers.

Policy Conundrums

Reproductive and genetic therapies also will pose difficult policy problems, often complicated by ideology.

In October 1999, a team of surgeons under Joseph Bruner at Vanderbilt University in Nashville successfully operated on a 21-week fetus in the womb to prevent brain damage from spina bifida, which had been diagnosed from an ultrasound scan. In spina bifida, the vertebrae fail to grow closed around the spinal cord, often resulting in inability to walk and other neurological disasters. The operation forestalled the brain damage, although no surgery yet can cure the condition itself. But a dramatic photograph of the fetal hand grasping Bruner's finger added fuel to the fiery controversy surrounding abortion. To those who believe that the rights of "the unborn" outweigh those of their mothers, the image made the fetus appear even more human and important.

The argument can only grow more heated and bizarre as science pushes the time of fetal viability back toward fertilization. When new techniques of lifesaving fetal surgery or complex genetic therapy become available, will states with "pro-life" legislatures pass laws forcing mothers to use these procedures rather than abort an unviable fetus or simply allow it to die? Both the therapy and the new life (often requiring costly extended care) will entail financial burdens. Will lawmakers force the expense upon even the poor? Or will they make taxpayers foot the bill? Any choice will be controversial.

The concept of informed consent takes on new dimensions,

too. Do persons-to-be have some sort of "right to nonexistence" if medical treatment saves their lives, only to leave them facing decades of disability and hardship? Will some of them turn to the courts for compensation? In France, such a "wrongful birth" suit (apparently the first) was recently decided for the plaintiffs—the parents and their 17-year-old son, born deaf, retarded, and partially blind after doctors and a medical laboratory missed a rubella (German measles) infection in the mother, thus depriving her of knowledge that would likely have prompted her to choose abortion.

The more sophisticated genetic design becomes, the worse the informed-consent paradoxes will be. For example, geneticists have discovered that the longest version of the D4DR gene on chromosome 11 diminishes the responsiveness of neurons in certain parts of the brain to dopamine, the so-called accelerator or arousal neurotransmitter. This helps produce what some psychologists call a "minimizer," someone whose interior responses to stimuli are phlegmatic. Such a person tends to seek novelty and adventure, racing cars or scaling mountains, as a way of getting the kind of dopamine rush that others get from less risky pursuits.

In 1996, when the long D4DR's effects were discovered, news anchors called it the "curiosity gene." The following year, when a statistical link between the long D4DR and heroin addiction was found, it became, with similar oversimplification, the "junkie gene."

Suppose, in the future, that a child with the long D4DR is born to parents who used genetic manipulation to preselect his traits. (They may have chosen the gene deliberately, or simply overlooked it among the welter of other options they weighed.) If the child in fact becomes a heroin addict, could he sue his parents, their genetic counselor, or the laboratory? How will the law decide to what degree DNA may account for the particular monkey on a particular back? If you think the courts are clogged now...

With issues like this in mind, scientists working toward genetic design in germ cells are thinking in terms of a two-stage process. The first stage would make the desired genetic change. The second would consist of two customized drugs, one to activate the gene, the other to deactivate it if it is no longer wanted. This approach not only solves the problem of prenatal informed consent but also ensures a robust aftermarket.

Some observers believe that the fears surrounding designer babies are exaggerated. They reason that the number of genes that combine to produce any one trait, multiplied by the blending of traits in a complete personality, multiplied again by the environmental and emotional influences that constantly modify internal biochemistry, all add up to a complexity that will be impossible to predict and control. It's a comforting thought, but it's also naive, and those who hold it excessively discount human technical ingenuity as well as the gargantuan research investment already made in the future of genetic modification.

At the very least, it should be possible to design *against* certain traits. For example, it will probably be feasible to modify the estimated dozen or so genes that influence sexual orientation. Dean Hamer's 1993 discovery of evidence for the existence of one of these, dubbed the "gay gene" in the popular press, was enough to add a seemingly scientific component to the antigay bigotry of the radio call-in opinion giver Dr. Laura Schlessinger. (She calls homosexuality a "biological error.") There will be lots of customers for sexual-orientation genetic therapy among those who gravitate to such teachers. If it works, will that be a good thing? Do we want a world in which sexuality (and perhaps the myriad cultural and social implications that historically go with it) is controlled by parental fiat?

Taking over such decisions ourselves by means of choices made in the genetic marketplace could lead us to change ourselves in self-defeating ways. Suppose, for example, we decided to selectively acquire for our children traits like optimism and trust, which work in a relatively stable, peaceful, nonexploitative world; by placing an order for them in our genetically tailored offspring, it might be possible to sweeten the personality of the entire human race. To anyone who has ridden the New York City subway this might seem like a good thing. But what if conditions change and we suddenly need more doubt and suspicion for a harsh environment? Will we have bred ourselves into a corner?

In terms of the human future, the commercial dynamic might be worse than biotechnology's attractiveness to tyrants. Retail eugenics could accomplish what the racialist regimes of history failed to achieve. All parents want easy, happy lives for their children—and themselves. If van Gogh's peculiar epilepsy is routinely cured, will anyone ever see the way he did again? Tendencies toward gender-bending, bookishness, lust, or defiance of authority might well be bred out. What if all types of quirky, nonlinear artistic vision come to be seen as curable defects? How would millions of such decisions by sane people be any different *in cumulative social effect* from one eugenic decision imposed on a nation by a tyrant?

Get a Head with Biocomputing

Research neurologists expect genetic medicine to make people's brains work better, far beyond the power of today's "smart

THE TERRIBLE GIFT

drugs." Changes to neuronal genes or their expression should enhance speed of association, math aptitude, possibly even such elusive traits as facility with metaphors or musical sensitivity. A research team led by the Oxford University geneticist Anthony Monaco has found the first of several genes that hardwire the planum temporale region of the brain for language. This discovery might be a gateway to learning more about the relationship between brain and mind (that is, structure and function), as well as to the creation of products for improving linguistic ability.

That gateway already has begun to open. In 1999, the Princeton neurobiologist Joe Z. Tsien modified a gene that encodes part of one type of nerve-cell receptor in the hippocampus–the brain structure in which memories are formed (though not stored)–of mice so as to increase the neuron's readiness to absorb calcium. This receptor conducts calcium ions into the cell, priming it to send an impulse onward in response to incoming signals from other neurons.

Tsien's "Doogie" breed of mice (named after TV's precocious Doogie Howser, M.D.) learn faster, apparently by forming memories more readily, and they have more curiosity than other mice, as measured by six standard tests of animal intelligence. Moreover, this is enhancement of healthy young brains, not restoration of declining old ones. There is no reason to believe that the same magic cannot be wrought in humans.

The real question, as Dr. Tsien wisely cautions, is what the trade-offs are. Will memory boosters make our heads overflow with too much data? In the fifties, the psychologist A. R. Luria studied a Russian who performed feats of memory as a stage act; the man said he often found it hard to concentrate under the rain of irrelevant details flooding his consciousness.

The whole field is yet another opportunity for "medical quickery." The annual $250 million sales of ginkgo biloba barely hint at the potential market for a definitive memory or intelligence drug. Will genetic razzle-dazzle lead us to neglect even more than we do already the simplest way to enhance learning ability: improving schools?

Genetic drugs are only one facet of research into ways to medically enhance human intelligence. We're in the process of launching an entirely new computer industry: biocomputing, which will use organic materials—including DNA and living cells—as computers, as well as connecting computers directly to plants, animals, and people. The resulting entities will be part living, part machine, like the cyborgs of science fiction.

Some seminal work in this field is being done by bioengineers at Bell Labs and Syracuse University. Using light-sensitive proteins derived from a common marine bacterium, they're building prototype blocks of "data jelly," storage units with a memory capacity of at least 10 gigabytes per cubic centimeter. Less than two decades after William Gibson wrote about brain plug-ins in his novel *Neuromancer,* it is no longer pure science fiction to envision a protein cube connected via biowire to the human hippocampus from a tiny "memory aid" tucked behind the ear. (But when the storage medium changes yet again, will our pasts be stuck on Betamax in a DVD world?)

In 1997, Jay Groves and fellow researchers at Stanford invented an artificial membrane that connects tissue to silicon chips. It gives cells biochemical feedback that makes them think they're touching other living cells. In the near term, this advance will lead to cell-array test chips much like gene-array chips. Thousands or millions of different receptor-bonding sites on a chip will induce blood cells, for example, to sort themselves into positions where electrical signals they generate can give an immediate readout of red and white cell counts. Such chips could do thousands of tests for leukemia or AIDS in the time it now takes to do one.

Conversely, by programming electrical impulses the other way, from chip to cells, or by shunting metered amounts of chemicals via microtubules through the synthetic membrane, researchers will be able to perform experiments on individual cells (drug efficacy tests, for example) and obtain instantaneously tabulated results.

Similar chips will use natural and artificial cells as sensors to test for environmental pollutants, mine gases, hospital infections, and chemical warfare toxins. Living Band-Aids will analyze a wound, sensing the type of damage and infecting bacteria, then secrete the proper healing enzymes and antibiotics.

In the somewhat more distant future, these tissue-silicon interfaces will lead to sensory prostheses much more powerful than the nonliving eye and ear implants currently under development. By about 2005, bioengineers hope to develop prototypes of implants to replace areas of the hippocampus damaged by epilepsy or Alzheimer's disease, and spinal cord bridges for seamless repair of paraplegia.

The same research will lead directly into the realm of sensory-upgrade modules for enhanced human capabilities, in the mode of TV's $6 million man. The applications might begin with add-ons for infrared or telescopic sight, superacute expanded-frequency hearing, or a doglike sense of smell. In other words, our scientific instruments will begin to migrate inside us.

So will our computers. DNA has been shown to be a semiconductor of electricity. Like silicon, it can be doped, alloyed with small amounts of catalysts to change its electrical properties, much the way a hint of a drug can dramatically alter consciousness. DNA strands can be plated with gold or silver to make nanowires of efficient copperlike conductivity. Researchers at the University of Saskatchewan recently found that zinc, nickel, or cobalt ions can fill the spaces between the rungs of the DNA ladder so as to conduct electricity while retaining the molecule's unique structural connectivity. This opens the way in the near future to self-reading probes for gene and drug testing, and to self-assembling nanostructures and biocircuitry later on.

Early research thus has proved the feasibility of building computers out of DNA. Of course, such computers may be subject to DNA's faults. Manic mutated programs might run amok like cancer cells. But DNA computers will have major advantages. They will be orders of magnitude smaller and faster than today's etched-silicon-chip designs, will use less power and produce less heat, and will run software that fixes its own bit rot (bugs caused by decay of the medium) using genetic self-repair processes.

Furthermore, DNA-based computing may be more versatile than silicon-based computing. The latter can handle only digital operations directly—manipulating discrete bits of 1 or 0—on or off. DNA is good at bits (the genetic code is a 4-bit digital system), but DNA is also well suited for analog computing, a world of curves, gradations, mixed results, and fuzzy logic. The structure of DNA is not limited to the double helix. DNA would be perfect for constructive computing, building unplanned molecular assemblies according to programmed rules from a library of elementary shapes—rings, balls, lattices, Möbius strips, and other geometric forms.

Some labs have done preliminary work on harnessing the shape-shifting structures of proteins, vastly more complex than DNA. Biochemists envision autonomous DNA factories running molecular motors to build completely artificial soft machines—

life forms like nothing in nature. The first stage of this industry might be drug-producing microbes to counterinfect patients against disease. Someday hybrid nanobots might scour away arthritis damage and deliver regenerative enzymes to grow and protect new cartilage.

Other researchers are making silicon-chip replicas of the small, well-mapped brains of the fruit fly, the sea slug, and the roundworm. They hope to learn how evolution has packed so much processing power into such limited circuitry and why brains—even simple ones—deal so much better than current computers with unexpected or confusing input. This replication of natural brains will link with the design of genetically engineered cells to grow customized neuron arrays as computers—in other words, artificial brains.

It will also lead to a deeper level of integration of other types of computers with the human body and brain. Inorganic switching molecules and conductive carbon nanotubes are small enough to build subcomputers inside protein molecules. As this technology matures, assemblies much more powerful than today's supercomputers could be small and cheap enough to be woven into clothing.

Why would you want supercomputers woven into your shirts? No one can say just yet. Perhaps they could listen in to your brain waves and offer help for the problems weighing on your mind. Perhaps they could monitor your vital signs and make menu suggestions based on your nutrient deficiencies. In any case, wearing a shirt like that, you'd always have someone to talk with.

Here comes more science fiction, rapidly turning into fact. The Defense Advanced Research Projects Agency is funding chip implants in monkey brains with the goal of using brain-wave sensors attached to the scalp to let soldiers run a robot, or pilots fly a plane, by *thinking* about what they want it to do. Likewise, paraplegics might use their minds to direct motors attached to their limbs. From there, it's easy to envision superfine muscle coordination for fighter pilots or Ping-Pong players, microconnected to their control yokes and paddles. Whole new sports based on thought-directed, motion-amplifying robot armor might fill tomorrow's satellite channels.

Future neural interfaces may include adjunct processors to add digital computing speed to the brain's unequaled analog powers of association and creativity. Temporary, replaceable implants of entire databases will be sold for specific financial, technical, or literary jobs. Say you want to write a book about genetics. Plug in (swallow?) a module with details of all gene research to date, and instead of looking it up, you can "remember" it.

We foresee a rather large market in detailed memories of college courses you never took, books you never read, and hot nights that someone else spent with various hunks and sylphs. Yes, these fantasies are already in the works. Berkeley experimenters have taken their first, blurry look through the eyes of a cat, achieved by hooking electrodes to 177 neurons in its thalamus. Eventually some unemployed young actor with a model girlfriend will become the first to rent out his sensory cortex. Imagine a direct-feed mind-cam, sending you telesensory experiences over your brainstem Netlink.

There's little question that the difference between natural and artificial intelligence is going to narrow, if not disappear altogether. Increasingly, the question will become: Which of these cascading more or less living gadgets will you spend your disposable income on?

Or to put it another way: Where the hell are we headed?

People Who Seed People

Sometime in the next five years—perhaps even by the time this sentence is printed—a private, well-funded, but somewhat fly-by-night lab will announce its success in cloning a human being from an adult (clones of human embryos have already been made).

Who will claim this breakthrough? It might be the secret Clonaid lab set up in an undisclosed nation by the Raelians, a French and Canadian UFO society founded on the belief that the human species was originally cloned by aliens. Clonaid's ultimate goal is to enable gay partners to have genetic children, but their first project is to re-create an American couple's dead daughter. They announced the start of the attempt in October 2000, claiming a list of 50 surrogate mothers willing to incubate the large number of trial embryos needed for eventual success.

The breakthrough will proceed in secret, of course. The ethical questions around cloning are too hot for the big granting institutions. Indeed, human cloning is already legally prohibited in the European Union and the United States.

Certainly there are technical obstacles to overcome before cloning of humans can become routine. At present, it usually takes hundreds or thousands of attempts to get one cloned animal embryo, most cloned embryos die early in development, and those that survive to full term die at birth at least twice as often as fetuses conceived normally. At every stage, clones manifest an enormous incidence and variety of genetic defects. Some cloned embryos that died soon after fertilization have even been found to consist entirely of cancer cells! As yet, scientists have few clues as to what goes wrong, or why their attempts occasionally succeed. Experiments with mice so far indicate that clones from out-bred, or genetically diverse, strains or from stem cells are more likely to be viable than those from inbred mice or fully differentiated cells.

Dolly, the famous cloned sheep, was born with a reduced number of telomeres. Apparently as a result of this, at last report she is indeed aging prematurely and is unhealthily obese. This syndrome may mean that all clones that, like her, are made from postembryonic cells will be subject to premature aging, a genetically reduced life span. However, as noted in Chapter 7, clones of cows made by a different process, using embryonic cells, were bequeathed *extra* telomeres, possibly lengthening their lives.

Eventually, as the technical issues are resolved, human cloning will take root. Ineffectually braked by stopgap laws that vary from country to country, the industry will develop first in "bio-havens" that choose cash over restrictions, the techno-medicine equivalent of offshore banking havens like the Cayman Islands.

A series of cloning techniques for creating parts of people will prepare the way for public acceptance. Cloning of partial DNA sequences and bacterial cell lines are already long-established laboratory techniques. In animal husbandry, cloning is being developed for the ultimate in purebred strains yielding the biggest eggs and the juiciest meat. It will be used to standardize and stabilize genetically modified foods—low-cholesterol eggs and beef, for example. Scientists are already using cloning to replicate lab rats and monkeys for precise study of genetic additions and subtractions. And PPL Therapeutics of Scotland has cloned pigs as a step toward providing human-friendly assembly-line organs for transplants.

In February 2000, the European Patent Office in Munich granted the University of Edinburgh and Stem Cell Sciences of

Australia rights to a technique for cloning mammalian stem cells. It appeared that bleary-eyed patent examiners must have missed the phrase "including human cells," which was buried deep within the 235 pages of the application. Consequently, legal challenges to the patent have been filed by Greenpeace, Germany, the European Parliament, and hundreds of other groups and individuals, which may give examiners a chance to reverse their decision.

The "oops" explanation was called into question, however, by the subsequent discovery of a similar patent, granted more than a year earlier. In January 1999, Amrad, an Australian maker of genetically modified lab mice, received a patent covering a method of cloning stem cells to make embryonic hybrids of mice, sheep, pigs, goats, fish, and humans. The idea is eventually to produce disposable human-animal hybrids as organ banks. (The patent has since been sold to Chemicon, an American firm.)

European governments now are seeking laws to give them greater control over the patent office. In some contexts, we recoil from doing to people what we do to other species.

Initially, however, the Stem Cell Sciences process for cloning stem cells will be used to make an inventory of homogeneous natural stem-cell types from a variety of species, to be used for research. That is a compelling medical goal, and progress toward it already will be well along when opponents finish the procedures to invalidate the patent. Even if they succeed, the research will continue elsewhere. Organ-donor hybrids would save many lives, despite the instinctive repugnance that the idea produces.

Nor will borderless business be stopped by local or even national laws. Roslin Bio-Med of Edinburgh is a commercial offshoot of the publicly funded Roslin Institute, where Dolly the sheep was cloned. When California's Geron Corporation bought the company in 1999 it also acquired a British patent on a method of cloning human embryos—the American version of the patent applies only to nonhuman mammals.

The inexorable power of money will push back the ethical boundaries that today constrain the technology of cloning, bringing medical benefits but also unsettling social phenomena. Will the donor's relatives and friends expect a clone to be his or her exact duplicate? They're liable to be disappointed. Cyril, Cecil, Cedric, and Tuppence, four rams cloned by Dolly's creator, Ian Wilmut, were distinct in size, color markings, and temperament. Personalities of human clones are likely to vary remarkably because of different life experiences. That should lay to rest some of our fears about new Hitlers out of *The Boys from Brazil*, although some clone producers may try shaping the product after birth as well as before. (Think of the opportunities for religious or military indoctrination.) In any event, cloning should provide some interesting and original evidence related to the age-old nature-versus-nurture question.

The Hopeful and the Bizarre

Some of the possibilities of whole-human cloning are hopeful. It could provide biological children for single parents or infertile couples for whom in vitro fertilization has failed, or offspring who are exact genetic duplicates of children who have died or of other deceased loved ones. At least two billionaires have advanced the cause by funding research toward having beloved pets cloned. The best-publicized has been the Missyplicity Project, an effort by Mark Westhusin and his colleagues at Texas A&M University to clone Missy, a deceased dog owned by the project's anonymous Bay Area underwriters. The work is likely to have been successful by the time you read this. The project has spun off Genetic Savings & Clone, a company with both for-profit and nonprofit divisions devoted to cloning, respectively, DNA from pets and endangered species.

Genetic offspring for homosexual couples will become possible, maybe as early as 2003. The nuclear transplantation technique used to clone Dolly the sheep will be adapted to transfer the nucleus of a sperm cell into an egg whose nucleus has been removed, creating a "male egg" which can then be fertilized by another sperm. Lesbian sperm will follow. This development seems sure to be a major source of controversy in the next few years, but it could be among the most beneficial in terms of social acceptance of diversity.

Some potentialities will confer both benefit and harm, or will just be incomprehensibly weird. Clones of animals and humans with modified genomes could become a new art form—fantastic medieval bestiaries come to life. Organ replacement using stem-cell technology will involve a delay while the new organ is grown in the lab. What if you need one in a hurry? The wealthy may quietly contract for shadow clones, headless bodies with de-activated immune-tagging systems, grown in sterile bubbles to serve as organ trees, a ready supply of transplantables for family and friends. In return for the lives saved, will we ever get used to the horror-movie vision of semihuman things in vats? Or would such parts, having no connection with a neurocenter, be subtly defective?

Some of the prospects are unequivocally horrific: a new un-dercaste of slaves and servants? supersoldiers? mindless Mafia muscle? living sex toys? Would they be created with emotions or without? Would crucial mental functions be deleted to prevent organizing or rebellion? No doubt we'll see an array of . . . models? products? types? in a whole new high-stakes industry with rules and consequences we can't quite imagine yet.

CHAPTER 10

Silent Bombs

SCIENCE, LIKE CAPITALISM, IS AMORAL. Defiantly, proudly so. Many individual scientists and capitalists have personal moral values, of course, but the endeavors themselves have no widely accepted codes of ethics equivalent to medicine's Hippocratic oath.

As the sole aim of money is more money, so the sole aim of science (from the Latin *scire*, "to know") is more knowledge, a search for truth ideally unaffected by emotion or any notion of right or wrong. Furthermore, scientists, being human and ambitious, flock to the

"sweet problem," the "hot area," regardless of its potential destructive consequences.

The previous chapters were about the unpredictable, uninten-
tional evil effects of genetic medicine. This one and the next are
about the evil effects that are *entirely predictable* or *completely
intentional*. To assess them, we'll try to show medicine in its context within the larger field of biotechnology. By doing so, we argue that medicine shares responsibility for the social problems
that biotechnology is likely to engender—problems that the medical industry in its guises as both science and business would
rather ignore.

Our subject here is evil, harm inflicted on purpose or with
"reckless disregard," as the lawyers say. It's part of what Carl
Jung called the shadow, the hidden side of the human psyche,
which he pondered as Hitler's shadow loomed over Europe. In
the essay "What Christians Believe," C. S. Lewis called evil

the key to history. Terrific energy is expended—civilizations
are built up—excellent institutions devised; but each time
something goes wrong. Some fatal flaw always brings the
selfish and cruel people to the top, and then it all slides back
into misery and ruin. In fact, the machine conks. It seems to
start up all right and runs a few yards, and then it breaks
down.

Jung propounded a fundamental law of the dark side of the
human: It gets darker when you look away. This is why science
must not be governed entirely by scientists. Einstein said, "Rela-
tivity applies to physics, not ethics."

Thus, our next area of inquiry must be: What uses will evil
make of humankind's new genetic mastery?

Don't Try This at Home

Anyone can build a simple lab to genetically modify bacteria or plants for under $5,000. To work with viruses, insects, or small animals would cost more—perhaps $20,000 to $100,000 for a fairly complete setup directed toward a clear goal in one species. The basic equipment is readily available from supply houses, easily ordered by anyone with an academic or corporate letterhead. The procedures themselves are taught in colleges or published in scientific journals. In terms of apparatus, this isn't rocket science.

Of course, the prices we've discussed do *not* include clean rooms and redundant, fail-safe industrial containment systems. Unfortunately, the people and organizations interested in pursuing such work on the cheap, and on the sly, probably won't care much about safeguards.

Many biologists who are not preoccupied with promoting their own salable critters will admit, off the record, that even in the most advanced, legitimate genetic engineering labs no one *really* knows what they're doing yet. They know how to knock out a few genes and insert a few others; sometimes they even put them in a predetermined location. They can blenderize life forms and build rudimentary chromosomes from scratch. Sometimes they produce the forerunners of spectacular new products and medical treatments. It's all impressive enough by comparison with what was possible a decade or two ago.

But the areas of ignorance remain vast. Geneticists don't have the slightest idea why most mammals have about 3 billion base-pairs of DNA while salamanders have 50 billion and tiger lilies have 100 billion. They don't understand why humans economize with 23 chromosomes while crabs splurge on 250. There seems to be no rhyme or reason to the way these numbers vary among species.

We marvel at the amount of information contained in the human genome, which has as many "letters," base-pairs, as 800 Bibles. Our cells seem to use only 8 or 10 Bibles' worth, about 35,000 genes. Yet behold all the information that comes *out*— 100,000 proteins, and their thousands of folding patterns, and their place in cell structures, and their interplay in each cell as complex as a city, and the cooperative growth of 100 trillion cells into tissues, and tissue architecture into organs, and the integration of organs into a body and a mind, complete with instincts, the thousand blending traits of a whole personality, and so on and on. It seems as though 8 million Bibles wouldn't be enough.

But not only don't we know all the words, we can't really hum the tune yet. About 10 percent of the human genome is too repetitive to be sequenced with current methods, and similar areas in the genomes of other species are also unexplored. Researchers believe that these regions contain many of the control sequences that orchestrate the precisely timed riffs and silences of thousands of genes playing together to make the music of life. If one player in an orchestra falls a beat behind, those nearby, thinking they're at fault, may try to compensate in several different ways, and so the chaos spreads. Musicians call such a cascading dysfunction a train wreck. In genetics, it's called a deleterious mutation.

In a few years, we must anticipate scores of well-meaning scientific loners trying to cure diseases that have markets too small to generate a profit for the big players. Anticapitalist guerrilla geneticists will try to resist the commercialization of life by sabotaging the efforts of their corporate counterparts, but, working in haste and isolation, as they must, they may cause unintended harm of their own. And a third group, tomorrow's technological pranksters, will move on from computer viruses to genetic engineering, hoping to put their embedded tags on some nastier damage.

We have here an extremely volatile situation—a new science of enormous resources, vast ignorance, and low entry costs, with the power to invisibly make changes in our own bodies and in life all around us. The situation could blow up at any time. There's no question that genetic garage mechanics are going to release some newly engineered strains of life. Like natural mutations, most of the artificial ones will damage the organism and will die out. But evolutionary geneticists estimate that, even among spontaneous, random DNA changes, one out of a hundred or so confers a survival advantage. The percentage will probably be higher among those designed for viability.

Inevitably, a few of the unsanctioned mutants will be highly adaptive and invasive—a new kudzu, let's say, or perhaps a cold-adapted yeast that attacks trees during their winter dormancy. Such an organism might decimate northern forests by the time an eradication agent could be developed and used. Natural evolution might restore balance only after widespread initial devastation. If we're lucky, such outbreaks will be well-contained problems that won't directly affect humans. If we're unlucky, the damage could be much worse.

New Weapons from the Lab

Many gene hackers will be absorbed by mainstream industry, but some will graduate from basements to better-financed secret labs. Genomic technology is likely to spawn new forms of terrorism using weapons with a wider radius than explosives. With no bomb bits or upload links to trace, most of the villains may never be found. We might not even know for months or years that a genetic bomb has gone off.

Not all backroom players are poor. The potential for major mischief from minor-league governments, holy warriors, and criminal cartels is truly disturbing. In 20 years of secret work after signing the 1972 treaty outlawing development of germ-warfare agents, the Soviets went ahead and made weapons out of smallpox, pneumonic and bubonic plague, and the Ebola and Marburg viruses. They amassed a genetic database of three thousand strains of anthrax, some of them adapted to specific delivery systems and recombined with genes from other bacteria to make them immune to any known vaccine. Before the Gulf War, Iraq developed munitions using botulism and gangrene. Modern global travel patterns mean that infection of just a few dozen people with a slow-acting, highly contagious, untreatable pathogen could sicken hundreds of millions throughout the world in a few months, an appalling scenario that we dramatized in the Introduction to this book. A strain of tuberculosis from the Soviet Union has reportedly appeared in New York City.

If medicine becomes a huge genetic paint-by-numbers kit, what kind of pictures will we get in a world of Serb and Croat, Hutu and Tutsi, Ku Klux Klan and Farrakhan? White South African biologists working under the direction of Dr. Wouter Basson tried to make a biopoison aimed at the melanin levels in black skin, to be sold in beer or spread by vaccination. Apartheid fell before they finished, but they gave their work-in-progress to Israel's chembio center at the Institute for Biological Research at Nes Tziyona, near Tel Aviv. The common Semitic ancestry of Jews and Arabs may slow the development of ethnically targeted genetic warfare in the Middle East, but Israeli researchers have found a gene cluster common among Iraqis that could serve as a possible target for an air- or waterborne virus.

There are four known Russian germ-war centers that are closed to outsiders, and there are half a dozen others at which research is being funded by American agricultural and military agencies. They include Vector, a Siberian virus lab, and Obolensk, a huge bacteria factory 50 miles south of Moscow. Ostensibly our taxes go there only to fund work on antidotes to bioweapons, and to inoculate underpaid Russian scientists against bribes from the other nations known to be working on biological arsenals: China, Egypt, Iran, Iraq, Israel, Libya, North Korea, Syria, and Taiwan.

We'll see whether this strategy works. There may be excess germ-gene talent that even fistfuls of U.S. dollars can't soak up, and there has never yet been a weapon that was purely defensive. The United States regards itself as uninvolved in biological-warfare research because the attack side of its program is overtly directed only against prohibited drug plants, but our government classifies anticrop weapons as offensive when wielded by others.

In the future, diseases that jump readily from animals to humans, such as swine flu, may be modified to produce epidemics that destroy both people and their food supply, while remaining unrecognizable as hostile attacks. Crop killers look like a growth market, too. Iraqi scientists have done extensive work on wheat smut, a crop-destroying fungus that also produces trimethylamine gas, an explosive that can blow up granaries. Before 1972, the United States devised some ingenious delivery systems for biological weapons, such as infected turkey feathers dispersed by bombs like those used for blanketing an area with propaganda leaflets.

American biowarfare proceeds today as an offshoot of the drug war. Scientists at the Agricultural Research Service in Beltsville, Maryland, and at a British center that has recruited unemployed Soviet bioweapons brains are trying to use genetically engineered fungi and viruses to render cannabis, coca, and poppies extinct. Test versions of the pathogens are now being or soon will be sprayed in Uzbekistan, Kazakhstan, Peru, Colombia, and Florida. The obsessive desire to enlist microbes as drug police could easily yield modified plant diseases with unintentionally catholic tastes.

Even absent new developments, the currently stockpiled germ weapons represent a threat at least as grave as garage-sale nuclear weapons—and much easier to hide. For the future, medicine may not be able to prevent a DNA arms race, but surely its leaders have a duty to oppose any government's use of the weaponry for its own agendas.

Accidents Will Happen

Some results of biotech medicine will never be announced in press kits. As with any new technology, accidents are guaranteed. And in a capitalist system, the cost of efforts to prevent or repair accidents is always weighed against the bottom line. Thus, some level of error and destruction is always considered financially tolerable—and therefore inevitable.

There are plenty of precedents for these profitable atrocities. The capitalist hero Lee Iacocca presumably read the crash-test reports written by the Ford engineer Harley Kopp in the early 1970s and apparently decided it would be cheaper to pay off a few hundred Pinto widows than to retool the production line. And it was–$100 million cheaper.

Bhopal was an accident of negligence compounded by contempt for the inhabitants of its Third World location. In another case, Monsanto in 1998 sold cotton seed in parts of India without mentioning that it was a genetically engineered test batch. The crop failed in an environment where one harvest is all that stands between many Indian families and starvation. At least 112 ruined farmers committed suicide in the aftermath of their crop's failure, making this biotechnology's first known fatal "accident."

Closer to home, birth control has been a fertile field for technological accidents. The story of the intrauterine birth control device is a classic example of waste and suffering caused by dollar-driven medical development. Of numerous possible designs for a contraceptive IUD, the Dalkon Shield was first and foremost to market. Safety testing had disclosed the danger of uterine infection. Nonetheless, the appliance was sold in the United States from 1972 to 1974, with considerable profit to its maker, A. H. Robins. After the Dalkon Shield was banned by the FDA, surplus inventory was dumped overseas via the Agency for International Development. All told, 195,000 of 2.8 million American users eventually sued for damages. For several years, legal foot dragging and concealment of the early safety reports limited the company's losses from lawsuits to amounts made up by returns on Robins's invested profits.

Finally, in 1989, after a 15-year legal battle, a $2.5 billion fund was established to compensate the injured. Furthermore, a buyout of Robins stock at $29 a share was arranged as part of the legal settlement; when the company declared bankruptcy four years earlier, the market price had been $8. The stock sale netted an estimated $350 million for the Robins family.

That's nearly $3 billion in total costs attributable to the Dalkon Shield. These costs were paid in several ways: through higher prices to customers and lower dividends to investors of American Home Products, which bought the Robins stock; through higher premiums paid by customers of Aetna, Robins's insurer, which paid $500 million into the compensation fund, plus miscellaneous damage awards; through taxes, which covered court costs and most of the damage fund; and through higher health-care prices due to the ripple effect on liability insurance for other medical products.

The $3 billion amount does not include lawyers' fees, victims' medical expenses, or Robins's prebankruptcy profits. The actual total may have been over $5 billion. Even that number doesn't include damages to Third World women, always heavily discounted.

Aside from suffering, the worst part of the whole fiasco is that a promising birth control method that could have been developed safely has been tainted and lost. Sometimes the much-touted alchemy of the profit motive turns gold into lead.

The new biotechnology is being developed in a business climate that is, if anything, more profit-oriented than ever. How can we not expect more episodes like the Dalkon Shield affair?

Fallout on the Farm

Our rush to redesign life to our liking may involve unexpected costs to our physical health. One of the chief early aims of plant biotechnology is to engineer high levels of natural pesticides into crops, so that farmers can cut down on artificial ones. Supposedly this will save money and perhaps even launch a second Green Revolution in the Third World. Few mention that the first

Green Revolution, beginning in 1964, benefited primarily agribiz landholders who could buy discounted fertilizers and pesticides for the fragile, high-yield strains of rice and other crops that were introduced at that time. If farmers now have to buy monopoly-priced seed every year or else face patent-infringement suits for saving and using their own seed, much of the putative savings will be illusory.

Moreover, most insecticides made by plants are carcinogenic to humans for the same reason artificial ones are: They damage DNA. But being inside the plant, they can't be washed off. Co-evolved natural levels of pest-killing chemicals are virtually harmless over normal life spans, but inducing crops to produce more of them may subject humans to cancer risks thousands of times greater than risks from chemical sprays, as the renowned carcinogen researcher Bruce Ames has been warning since the early nineties. That effect might nullify the benefits of the forth-coming advances in cancer treatment for which we have such high hopes.

Incorporating new poisons from unrelated species may exac-erbate the dangers, both by threatening consumers of the food and by damaging the ecological web. For example, there is evi-dence that the pollen of Bt corn, Monsanto's patented strain modified by adding a gene for *Bacillus thuringiensis* toxin, is killing off monarch butterflies. This may be an educational fore-taste of our own medicine.

The whole drive to develop genetically modified plants that produce their own pesticides is a classic case of a spiraling tech-nological feedback loop. Monoculture crops, with genetic varia-tion removed to enhance marketable characteristics, are notoriously vulnerable to pests and dependent on sprays. Now, unfortunately, plantings of monoculture crops have suddenly expanded, rising to half of American soybeans and a third of American corn since 1996. This trend may speed up evolution of resistant pest varieties anyway, worsening the very problem that pesticide genes were intended to solve—but also creating a market for a solution to the solution.

The Food and Drug Administration and the Department of Agriculture have shifted much of the safety burden onto the backs of farmers. For example, to forestall the appearance of resistant bugs, growers of Monsanto's Bt corn must plant a percentage of their acres in normal corn. They are asked to plant these "insect preserves" upwind, to prevent the Bt transgene from spreading into other corn types.

In crops grown on biodiverse acreage, which is still generally the norm in agrarian nations, hybridization can be expected to transfer any new gene into other plants and the ecosystem beyond. In their work on altered golf-course turfs, Scotts and Monsanto have found that pollen from grasses, which are much shorter than corn plants, spreads as far as a thousand feet. Herbicide immunity produced by traditional breeding methods has already spread from crops to some weeds. Many agronomists predict the same fate for Monsanto's Roundup-resistant gene, engineered into its Roundup-Ready plants as part of a single package to cover both the seed and the spray market. In fact, chemical traces of genetically engineered genes have recently been discovered in wild Mexican maize, an outrage in a country where for thousands of years corn has been synonymous with the life of the people.

Fear of gene-sprawl, the spread of engineered genes to other populations, has prompted attempts to get Monsanto to forgo using another of its patented gene products, known as Terminator. It renders crop plants sterile, thus enclosed, monopolized, and growable only from patented one-year seed. If fully deployed, the Terminator gene would drive most small farmers in poor lands to extinction and reduce the survivors everywhere to a kind of corporate serfdom. If the gene were to spread into the wild, it could sterilize other species and possibly drive them to extinction along with the animals that feed on them. In 1999, Monsanto said it would not use this genetic copy-protection device for now. Other companies hold patents on similar sterilizing genes, however.

In any case, relying on the consistency of breezes to prevent cross-pollination is ... it's hard to come up with a metaphor silly enough. Cats running a mail-sorter? Xerxes lashing the ocean with chains to save his fleet? Asteroid roulette?

It has also become the farmers' job to check for emergence of Bt-resistant pest strains. Thus they are being expected to do some of the seed companies' research for free. Monitoring so far has turned up no evidence of resistance, but five years is a short time for such evolution, even among insects. At this point, only the continued refusal of the European Union to knowingly import unlabeled genetically engineered grain is preventing the whole world from becoming an experimenters' lab.

What other kinds of biofallout can we expect to settle on us? Putting Brazil nut genes in soybeans to repel pests has increased yields, but it has also exposed people with nut allergies to increased risks, since soybeans can now serve as the Trojan horse for delivery of allergens to unsuspecting consumers. The danger is especially insidious because soybeans are an unlisted ingredient in many kinds of industrial food, from soup to ice cream. In retrospect, it seems like an obvious, easily foreseeable danger.

Add a dose of profit-driven concealment, and entirely new fields of work for medical investigators open up. The story of deception surrounding Monsanto's recombinant bovine growth hormone (rBGH) is a case in point. In 1994, after reviewing a Monsanto study that found no problems in rats fed rBGH, the FDA approved its use to stimulate higher milk production in dairy cows. (The agency then threatened to penalize dairies for telling customers if their cows produced milk *without* the stimulant.) In cows, rBGH raises blood levels of insulin-like growth factor 1 (IGF-1), which in turn stimulates milk production. In humans, high blood levels of IGF-1 are associated with much greater incidence of breast and prostate cancer. This rang alarm bells with many critics. In response, Monsanto pointed out that natural milk has IGF-1 in it (although that doesn't prove that the substance is healthy for humans). They also claimed that rBGH is safe because IGF-1 doesn't accumulate in a cow's body.

However, Canada has withheld approval of rBGH for at least two years of further study after doctors reviewing Monsanto data found a "previously unreported" effect: Nearly a third of the test rats had produced antibodies to IGF-1, proving that enough of the foreign hormone had entered their bloodstream after digestion to trigger a response from the immune system.

The Doomsday Cell

Genetic medicine and biotechnology promise to redefine the relationship of humans to nature from one of control to omnipotent manipulation. These technologies promise to be different from all previous technologies that have changed human life in three fundamental ways: *exponentiation, confluence,* and *autonomy.*

Computer scientists are well on their way to building systems that, if they don't reach true originative intelligence, will at least coordinate inputs well enough to achieve the sophisticated responses of instinct. Eventually, robots will become the new working class, and the poor will have no value even as cheap labor.

At the same time, nanotechnologists will be making microscopic machines to spec using single atoms and molecules as design components. Concurrently, biotechnologists will develop virtuoso skills at using genes to grow artificial biota. To fulfill their functions, many products of these industries will be given the ability to self-replicate. Such entities would, in effect, have a will to survive and multiply, whether or not they are conscious or "truly alive." Of necessity, they will evolve—become better at what they do—in response to selective pressures. Over time, such evolution will grow more efficient and speed up. This speedup of artificial biological evolution is what we mean by exponentiation.

Each of these industries will incorporate aspects of the others. Computational robotics will be applied to molecular engines, which will grow connections to all telecommunications media. Living cells will show nanobots how to reproduce, organize, and cooperate. The nanobots in turn will make biocells tougher and give them hands full of tiny tools. That's confluence.

Androids will begin using the Web to trade data for the factories they run. By then bacterial machines will be well established in our bodies, making drugs and performing housekeeping chores. Machines on both the macro- and microscopic levels will progress to designing the products and the production process for uses we specify. In other words, they will begin to develop culture, direct their own evolution, and interact with another species. In time, their purposes too will become their own. Behold, autonomy.

These changes will happen gradually, over decades. Each increment will occur because it represents an increase in efficiency and income for the owning corporation. Is it profit supremacy or natural selection? Does it matter?

Where do we humans fit in, in this all-too-possible future? Nowhere, actually. As George Dyson laid out the odds in *Darwin Among the Machines*, "In the game of life and evolution there are three players at the table: human beings, nature, and machines. I am firmly on the side of nature. But nature, I suspect, is on the side of the machines."

Among nanotech theorists this outcome is nothing new. It's called the "gray goo" problem. Bill Joy, the codeveloper of Unix and Java, gave it another look recently. First he found himself amazed at how naive even the best thinking about the danger seemed to him now, a decade after first reading. He cites Eric Drexler's proposal in *Engines of Creation* of a nanobot immune system for the biosphere, engineered to attack and destroy stray organisms escaping the labs. Apparently Drexler never thought of the idea that the shield might develop an autoimmune disease and attack the biosphere on its own—Gaia with leukemia.

As to the escapees, Drexler cites a few very simple examples of self-replicating molecular assemblers that might do us in. It will be only a few years now before designers of artificial chloroplasts achieve an improved version of photosynthesis, tripling or quadrupling chlorophyll's efficiency at turning light into food. Should "plants" containing these cells ever be released into the wild—by a careless night watchman or an overturned truck or an angry ex-employee—they will have an enormous competitive advantage over all previous foliage. Within a few years every plant on earth might be replaced by vegetation that no animal can digest.

It might not even take that long. Picture an omnivorous nanobot bacterium developed for those tough industrial cleanups. It develops a mutation in the gene that's supposed to kill it in the absence of a certain catalyst. With no natural enemies, it could wipe out all life on earth in less than a week.

Biotech medicine will offer us many gifts, both as individuals and as a society. Only a one-dimensional cynic would suggest that we should reject them all. But some of these gifts will be so inherently dangerous that we must somehow summon the will to renounce them before they are developed.

Who Bears the Risks?

At the moment, biotechnology enjoys "most favored industry" status among regulators. In 1992, almost two years before introduction of the FlavrSavr tomato, which was the first genetically modified (GM) food, Michael Taylor, then the FDA's deputy commissioner for policy, ruled that GM foods are inherently safe and need carry no informational labeling. In so doing, he ignored warnings from many of the agency's own scientists, as subsequently released internal papers prove. In fact, some FDA scientists warned that artificially inserted genes have a "unique" possibility of interacting in unforeseen ways with other genes to produce poisons found nowhere in nature. In 1989, an unknown toxic contaminant in a batch of tryptophan, an amino acid dietary supplement sold as a relaxant and sleep aid, killed 37 Americans and permanently injured 1,500 more. Some scientists have suggested that this debacle was the first GM food accident. Showa Denko K.K., the Korean company that manufactured the tainted shipment, was the first to do so using a genetically modified bacterium.

Deputy Commissioner Taylor, a lawyer, had represented Monsanto before he started to work in the government, and became the company's vice president for public policy afterward. This kind of revolving-door movement between business and government is commonplace, but in a complex, unproven field like biotechnology, such "round heels" regulation could end up hurting the industry along with the public.

Much of the burden of vigilance against potential dangers in the foods we eat is falling on the public. The European Union's grain-labeling requirement, together with a pledge by Gerber and Heinz not to use GM produce in their baby foods, has launched a market for companies that test products for genetic adulteration. The field is led by Genetic ID of Fairfield, Iowa, a company founded by John Fagan, a former NIH gene-therapy researcher. The USDA has responded by trying to persuade manufacturers to adopt some sort of "GM-free" labeling standard. Of course, it would be purely voluntary, backed by no compliance checks and providing no way of knowing which unlabeled products *do* include engineered biotics.

So far, the only speed bump on the road toward widespread genetic manipulation of foods has been produced by European concerns and the political impact of the 1999 Battle of Seattle. In November of that year, nonviolent protesters disrupted the World Trade Organization meeting sufficiently to induce delegates at the next meeting, in Montreal, to adopt the Biosafety Protocol, an exemption to WTO supersession of national law. The protocol allows member nations to refuse to import GM food without fear of trade sanctions. They may even do so as a precaution in the absence of persuasive scientific evidence as to harm or safety. The subsidiary Advanced Informed Agreement brings the principle of informed consent to food, giving signatory governments a right to know what's in their imports and how the ingredients have been manipulated.

Of course, it's clear that current rules represent only one stage in what is sure to be a complicated and drawn-out battle for control of this technological arena. In sorting through such disputes, we can expect about as much honesty and openness from Big Genetics as we got from Big Tobacco on the dangers of smoking. In the near absence of meaningful governmental and industrial vigilance, it will become part of medicine's duty, and our expense, to test our food for health risks.

And even gathering information is not without risk in the current economic and legal climate. In the looking-glass world of corporate law, the concept of proprietary data has come to mean that companies can literally own the truth. Revelation of facts, even when blowing the whistle to alert the public to a clear and present danger, may be considered "tortious [wrongful] interference in restraint of trade." Even if the argument doesn't stand up in every case, the multinational corporations that wield it can make the cost of doing legal battle against them prohibitively high.

How does this economic censorship work in practice? In 1997, two reporters for a Fox-TV station in Clearwater, Florida, did a story on Monsanto. Overawed by the company's reputation for gangland-style displays of courtroom muscle, management forced them to rewrite the story 83 times, then finally killed it, offering the reporters a total of $151,250 to quit their jobs and shut up.

In England, the *Ecologist* magazine planned to devote its entire autumn 1998 issue to an investigation of Monsanto—only to have the printer shred every copy rather than fight the company if it should bring suit under Britain's notoriously pro-business libel laws.

In *The Coming Anarchy*, the futurist Robert D. Kaplan takes a hard look beyond the First World economic boom of the 1990s. He sees a desperate planet, robbed of its real wealth by technology deployed under profit pressure without regard for life, then reduced to chaos by revolt and suppression. The terrorist atrocities of September 2001 seem at first glance to have more to do with religious extremism than revolt against injustice, but they clearly illuminate the vast reservoir of rage being created among the world's poor.

As they turn to the small screen to glimpse lifestyles of the rich and heinous, the majority of people on earth feel like Indians watching a Western. In January 2000, Ecuador tied the value of its unit of currency, the sucre, to the value of the American dollar. The move brought instant destitution to the poor and poverty to the middle class. In Quito, native people held a demonstration. They accosted everyone they found wearing a suit and tie, forcibly dressed them in traditional clothes, and made them join in ancient tribal dances for several hours.

In the United States, businesses reap $2.15 in profit for every dollar they spend on wages and benefits. Between 1995 and 2000, that ratio grew 16 percent, and it's much larger in our economic colonies. Workers of the world soon will have some surprising new reasons to unite, but we doubt that many protests will be as gentle and educational as the one in Quito. Do we enter the cost of the next round of revolutions under "Capital Expenses" or "Medical Losses"?

Will biotechnology bring dollar despotism to full fruition? Will medicine play the part of good German, or, in the name of its ancient social conscience, will it try to help create a more humane and inclusive society?

We are embarking on projects that can do great good if carried out with openness and caution, but they are being pursued within an investment-growth system noted for secrecy and reckless disregard for those whom it exploits. It's a recipe for disaster.

Everything Is Under Control

IN THE PREVIOUS CHAPTER, WE TALKED about some results of medical biotechnology that will obviously be evil. In this chapter, we'll discuss another danger: the role medicine will play in the erosion of human freedom—its impending contributions to the surveillance ethos and to the power of authoritarian control.

Of course, these medical "treatments" will be administered under the guise of ridding the body politic of villains or harmful chemicals. And terrorists certainly have created a legitimate need for better security measures.

The trouble is, it's often hard to keep police and governments from extending their concern with real dangers to encompass behavior that harms no one but which some may find objectionable. Then the quest for security becomes evil with a smiley face, and we risk turning medicine into the interrogator's doctor who's "only trying to help you"–Josef Mengele played by Marcus Welby. Such a cure is worse than the disease. How can we tell it for what it is, then? Perhaps the evangelist Matthew said it best: "By their fruits ye shall know them."

This chapter is a look at three such fruits in bud: genetic ID tracking, new fronts in the war on drug users, and techniques of mass mind control.

Your Genes in a Plastic Card

Knowledge is power, especially if your business is prophecy. Though they deny this, insurers will inevitably seek access to more and more detailed medical information about their clients. If laws restrict them, as a jumble of state and federal laws already do in part, they will offer discounts and better coverage in exchange for the data they seek. The result will be the same: a significant diminution of our already much-diminished sphere of privacy.

For their better policies, many insurers will require a unique health identifier (UHI), the medical ID card concept left over from Clinton's 1993 health-care speech, briefly discussed as a national mandate in 1997 and now revived as a tool against terrorism. This would be a standard piece of plastic containing an embedded fingerprint, a retinal scan, or a DNA sample to be matched to the bearer before any medical service is rendered–or firearms or airline tickets are sold. The 2000 Sydney Olympics pioneered the use of scannable gene-coded inks to distinguish genuine souvenirs from knockoffs. Each item was bar-coded with ink containing DNA from one of the athletes as a marker. In a few years, a DNA sample swabbed from the inside of your cheek may be bonded into most bank cards, credit cards, driver's licenses, and so on, replacing bar codes and magnetic strips as a means of foiling counterfeiters. Such a DNA identifier is the logical choice for medical ID cards.

Your UHI will give a doctor anywhere in the world instant access via the Internet to your medical history and genetic profile, to be used for customized treatment. Of course, once the coding gets linked to your Social Security number, other ID numbers, credit card numbers, phone number, street address, or e-mail address anywhere in the system, your medical records will be freely tradable among official and corporate servers.

If it were also applied to nonmedical transactions, a UHI could help protect a person from the burgeoning crime of identity theft. In 1999, a Margate, New Jersey, company called GeneLink became the first to establish a genetic ID registry. The customer gets a card sold over the Internet through insurance agents. It's backed by DNA samples and records stored anonymously and retrieved with a bar code. Such a card can't be used for identity theft without an inside accomplice.

A UHI coupled with a full-genome scan would let an HMO or insurance company set rates or deny coverage altogether on the basis of one's medical risk factors. Tied in with supermarket purchase-tracking "reward" cards, the UHI system could be used to raise premiums automatically for every bacon cheeseburger, mud pie, and six-pack you ingest. In 1997, the temptation for cost-minded medical police to enforce low-fat diets and exercise programs seemed so appalling to civil libertarians and food conglomerates alike that Congress and the administration quickly dropped the idea of creating a government-sponsored UHI. But free-market institutions will be happy to do the job for them.

The chief problem under any UHI setup will be deciding what uses of a person's genetic information should be legal and preventing unauthorized, illegal uses of it. Under the Kennedy-Kassebaum Health Insurance Portability and Accountability Act of 1996, people in group plans already have some protection from policy cutoffs and rate increases prompted by genetic test results. President Clinton gave a similar insurance provision to federal workers in 2000. Stronger laws to prohibit involuntary use of one's genetic data in all contexts may eventually be passed. They have nearly unanimous public support.

Genetic testing will raise many insurance issues, often putting privacy in conflict with coverage. Tests for breast- and ovarian-cancer-predisposing mutations in the two BRCA genes have been available since 1998. About a third of women at risk decline the tests for fear of losing their insurance, but, in general, insurers are paying for the tests to be done and are not getting to see the result, if they are done in the context of family history and counseling. They hope the tests will lead to more frequent checkups or preemptive surgery that could save them money on cancer treatment in the long run.

Of course, insurers do not want to pay for genetic "fishing expeditions" at the behest of the insured, especially since it can still cost a thousand dollars to check one gene. So they're being selective in what they agree to cover. But they do not take the same view when it comes to screening clients: In underwriting decisions, the trend is toward increasing use of genetic test results. In late 2000, the United Kingdom's Department of Health gave underwriters permission to use results of tests for Huntington's chorea. Insurers are expected to apply next for access to breast-cancer and Alzheimer's disease test findings. Since Britain's National Health Service provides universal coverage, results won't restrict access to medical services, but they will affect life insurance and mortgage qualifications.

During the next few years, several online companies will begin offering mail-in cheek-swab screening for a large array of disease and drug susceptibilities, using databases of SNPs that are relevant to human health. Price competition should quickly drive down the cost of this service, luring an increasing number of people to pay for testing out of their own pockets. In time, insurers may routinely pay for the tests, which would reveal opportunities for cost-saving preventive medicine, but such a practice will only intensify their desire to see the data.

There's little precedent for trying to prevent insurance companies from using genetic test results to set premiums or deny coverage. Treatment records have long been used in this way, a practice called *experience rating*, as opposed to the nearly defunct system of *community rating*, in which risk was shared equally and everyone in a region or age group paid the same premiums. Most gene tests, therefore, even those done anonymously, will be insurance-safe only if the patient does not act on the results and thereby create a treatment record. Furthermore, it's hard to see how government could prohibit genetic tests from being used for underwriting with the customer's okay in exchange for better coverage.

Rights and Wrongs of Data Privacy

The fundamental problem is that the idea of genetic privacy, like all privacy, runs counter to our entire commercial system, which considers medical records, like all personal information, to be just another database of potential customers, properly for sale to anyone. Rules announced by President Clinton in 1999 to take effect in 2002 seek to stop routine release and sale of electronic (but not paper!) medical records to banks, insurers, and marketers. (Police access will remain virtually unrestricted, so talking to one's doctor about illicit drug use will remain a potential hazard.) Some penalties are included in the new regulations, but infractions will be hard to prove, and, bowing to pressure from business, Congress has not granted a right to sue for damages from any discrimination that follows improper disclosure.

Much genetic information can be obtained indirectly anyway. For example, SNPs in a gene for cholesterol metabolism predict who will respond to the cholesterol-lowering drug pravastatin, but those are the same people most prone to high cholesterol levels and heart disease. Insurers need only pick out pravastatin users to redline this group of high-risk clients. Self-insured small-business employers who see their employees' medical bills can easily identify workers with expensive chronic conditions and find a pretext to fire them. Lawsuits arising from the first few such cases are in court as of this writing.

Moreover, there's no law against gathering genetic information on the sly—say, from urine tests for drugs. A test can be done even more stealthily. The law explicitly defines garbage as "abandoned property." Thus, your trash is fair game for cops, private eyes, or employers. A Styrofoam cup or used Kleenex will do quite nicely for a DNA sample. An envelope that you've licked will even have your corroborating address and fingerprints on it.

Genetic spying may find a place amid all the other forms of snoopery used by public and private investigators. But it may become increasingly unnecessary, too, as "nonmedical" DNA samples are routinely taken for identification purposes at birth, for license or credit applications, or upon arrest for even minor infractions.

It's an example of the double-edged sword of technology. Genetic databases will be as great an advance in crime solving as fingerprint databases were. Yet their potential for abuse is enormous. Such a gene base could be created by force of law, then sold by a cash-hungry government to businesses, as digitized driver's license photos already are by several states.

To some extent, handling of personal medical data may turn on individual choices and strategies. Employers hiring for certain jobs, such as work with hazardous chemicals, might require genetic tests and health policy surcharges or waivers. For other people, the question will be: How much privacy am I willing to give up for what level of medical security? Should I pay for genome screening out of my own pocket? Should I risk a promotion by betting that my insurer won't tell my boss about my risk of developing heart disease?

Increased linkage of computerized records makes these questions ever more complicated. A psychotherapist may paint my symptoms in the worst possible light to justify coverage for my treatment, but her report may come back to haunt me when I apply for life insurance or a government job. Many therapists in managed-care networks already avoid taking notes during sessions, lest they be forced to hand them over to reviewers in order to get monetary reimbursement for themselves or their clients from an HMO or insurer.

Now turn the question around and look at it from the public-policy standpoint. It might seem fair to penalize insurance customers for risky activities, like smoking or skydiving, but where do we draw the line? Drinking too much tends to cause disease and shorten life, but drinking a little, especially red wine with meals, helps protect against heart disease. Will we all get federal monitoring chips to assess our safety levels, with insurance rates adjusted monthly on the basis of the readouts?

The ethical underpinnings of these questions came into focus for many people in 1995, when the legendary baseball star Mickey Mantle, a decades-long alcoholic, needed a new liver. The procedure would cost $400,000, and with organs in short supply, giving Mantle a liver would inevitably mean that someone else would not receive one. Some asked whether Mantle's alcoholism—an inherent weakness if not a choice—shouldn't lessen his claim to such valuable medical resources. On what basis should we judge an individual's "worthiness" to receive treatment? And what role, if any, should a person's own culpabilities play in that judgment?

We think the only sensible answer is that, in the eyes of law and medicine, all lives must be considered equally valuable. If services must be rationed, let it be done by medical criteria applied evenhandedly to all, and then, if supply is still short, by some sort of lottery. Of course, that's an ideal that ignores the power of money. And would we really want to prosecute a rich man for buying health care outside the system to save his own life, or his wife's, or his child's? Still, to keep a residue of public trust, government must keep medicine from violating the ideal of equal treatment too flagrantly.

No right is absolute, and this principle should probably apply to DNA privacy as well. There may be a valid duty to disclose one's genetic profile to a child or a prospective spouse, for example. Sperm and egg banks will almost certainly require genome scans, but must they maintain long-term contact with donor and recipient to cover liability for genetic problems that later technology might reveal? Should a doctor be required to breach confidentiality if a test on a female patient shows that the woman's sister also is at high risk of ovarian cancer and the patient declines to share the information? What if the patient herself would rather not know? Can she sue either for being told or for not being told? Does the answer change if she develops terminal cancer that might have been caught by a timely warning?

Such questions are morally important, but they may become practically irrelevant as our zone of privacy shrinks. The transparency of our lives as data will continue to change the marketplace, often in unexpected ways.

How Useful Will Genetic Screening Be?

Will genetic screening actually yield enough prophetic power over multifactor ailments to nip great swaths of disease in the bud? That's still a very big question.

Some statistical and epidemiological evidence suggests that atherosclerosis, cancer, and most other untamed diseases are triggered by undiscovered bacteria and viruses—although their development is still influenced by a multitude of well-documented genetic, environmental, and lifestyle factors. The recent discovery of a bacterium that causes stomach ulcers lends weight to this argument. If this theory of unknown disease agents is correct, the difficulty of prediction is about to increase.

Genetics itself is a lot more complicated than the predictors might wish. Some mutant genes make extra copies of themselves in each cell division, knocking out more and more healthy genes in a way that cannot be foreseen. Other genes are gender-marked, causing disease if inherited through one sex but not the other. Some mutations develop and spread via genes contained in mitochondria, the cells' energy plants, which are completely outside the chromosomal system. And once in a while, a viable zygote forms with both sets of chromosomes donated by one parent—a natural clone. Aberrations like these add more silt to waters that statistically are already very muddy.

There's no question that genetic screening will help protect people against diseases caused by single-gene defects. The approach was dramatically vindicated in the first five people to have their stomachs removed to prevent a rare, deadly stomach cancer caused by a gene that could be screened for. All five had early tumors undetectable by other means.

At this point, it seems likely that some people who submit to genetic screening for more common illnesses will get relatively clear-cut forecasts—"an 80-percent lifetime chance of heart disease," for example, along with graphs of other risks. But given the complex interactions among thousands of genes, germs, toxins, and life factors, the readout for many may be no more helpful than "Maybe you will, maybe you won't."

Since everyone has at least a few dozen "abnormal" genes, broadband disease prediction may be too unreliable to be cost-effective as a basis for job or insurance discrimination. A finding of "no bad heart genes" might even encourage folk to skip the workouts and eat all the butter they want, moving them into the high-risk group after all. Even if genetic tests do become widely and accurately predictive, many people may opt to live in blissful ignorance rather than suffer anxiety or avoid the very things they enjoy most. Physicians already report surprise at patients' lack of interest in testing for the gene that causes nonpolyposis colo-rectal cancer.

In the short term, questions of whether to gather, reveal, or conceal one's genetic information will be one more high-pressure personal choice. The leverage that genetic testing will give em-ployers and insurers could lead to one more option—a black mar-ket in cash-off-the-books health care. While more honest in some ways, it would be subject to its own styles of abuse.

In the long run, even modest gains in medical prophecy, com-bined with consumer hunger for nontherapeutic medicine—medi-cine geared to retooling, not curing—doom the present insurance approach. On the personal level, the demands of schools, em-ployers, banks, mortgage lenders, adoption agencies, motor vehi-cle bureaus, tenure committees, landlords, governments, the military, and the police probably will make genetic information a standard part of every résumé and disclosure form, no more pri-vate than job history, rap sheet, or net worth statement. On the social level, genetic medicine seems likely to be dragooned into serving more sinister agendas of control.

New Drugs to Make War Against

This book isn't the place to delve in any detail into the evils wrought by the war on drugs. Entire books could be, and have been, devoted to an analysis of the whole sorry history. Among the destructive *medical* consequences of our hysterical reaction to psychoactive drugs are these:

- Driven by fear of chemically induced pleasure, the drug warriors take cheap, safe euphoriants first from the people and then from their doctors—as typified by the ongoing fight over medical marijuana, which is forbidden despite being, in terms of overdose potential, by far the safest drug known, legal or illegal.
- Counting the costs of narco-police, propaganda, judges, lawyers, prison builders, guards, soldiers, sprays, choppers, rats, and bureaucrats, plus vastly inflated prices for the drugs themselves, plus taxes and GDP that are eliminated with arrestees' jobs and careers, we pay an estimated $500 billion a year for the Dope War. Even so, despite rants about the "scourge," we can't seem to afford much help for most of the people fighting real problems of addiction. As many observers have ruefully noted, "The poor go to jail; the rich go to Betty Ford."
- Between 2 million and 3 million Americans are in jail. About half of them are drug prisoners. The war breaks up nearly 1 million American families every year, often permanently removing children from parents without any evidence of child abuse. The medical costs that result downstream from this process are hard to quantify, but no one can argue that it conduces to health.
- The Dope War increases damage and medical costs from the substances themselves. Under prohibition, drugs must be concentrated to save space and make concealment easier. The result is substances that are more potent, with

smaller margin for error in dosage. Furthermore, the war lets careless and deceitful manufacturers flourish, producing more medical problems. Thus many if not most of our 9,000 annual overdose deaths are caused by contaminants and uncertainty about dosage.

- The money at stake in the illegal business produces about half of the murders in the United States, just as it did during alcohol prohibition. Today that's another 15,000 needless deaths every year, plus many more battlefield injuries and their medical costs.
- A substantial minority of AIDS cases must be blamed on the drug war, inasmuch as the fear of encouraging heroin addiction prevents access legally to sterile syringes.

These medical costs are bad enough, but what about the intangible nonmedical costs, like the snitch culture, erosion of the Bill of Rights, use of prisoners for slave labor, and racist inequities in enforcement of the laws? Combined with the trend toward permanent denial of voting rights to felons, the last amounts to a new poll tax to disenfranchise African Americans.

When courting Third World politicians, the war's generals often talk about "reducing the market for drugs through education." Yet no one seems to have a clue what it is about modern life that creates such demand. The market will not only remain; it will increase as urban daily life becomes ever more complex and pressured for most people.

One of the side effects of genetic medicine will be to open up new fronts in the Dope War. Pharmacogenomic discoveries will yield higher highs, faster speeds, deeper nods, and more ecstatic ecstasies, all synthesized truer than ever to diverse genetic needs and receptor sites, with gentler morning-after rebounds. Candy and cosmetics makers have been among the first subscribers to genetic databases, to tune their products to the SNPs of human smell and taste. The market will cater to variants of mental taste, too, whether or not the law affords them equal protection.

Given the stress levels of modern life, we predict a growing escape market for pure side effects—drugs that simply mess you up, and do it so thoroughly that a two-week bender will seem by comparison like a sojourn in a seaside Zen retreat. Repair bills for these are likely to be enormous.

Since drug prohibition generates profits that turn little gangs into multinational cartels, it would be naive to expect all the suppliers of tomorrow's new highs to show up on NASDAQ. Even if the initial research is proprietary work funded by an aboveboard corporation, the recipe for a drug can often be pilfered or pieced together from tangential articles by scientists who don't want their names lost behind a corporate patent. And molecules can be analyzed and back-engineered. Numerous rebel chemists will be happy to do so, and they'll be able to come up with their own designs as well. Then it's easy for other labs to make the product.

A hint of one of the new black markets in drugs may be coming from the sports world. Endurance athletes are beginning to use perfluorocarbons (PFCs). Developed for use as a form of emergency replacement blood when whole blood is unavailable, PFCs have five times the oxygen-carrying capacity of hemoglobin, giving marathoners and cyclists the same kind of advantage that has made anabolic steroids indispensable to strength athletes and bodybuilders. The International Olympic Committee has added PFC metabolites to its test list, so the old cat-and-mouse game—train with drugs, flush for the meet—seems about to expand.

Stratified societies based on anguish and the threat of physical pain always want to supervise painkillers. The Opium Wars, in which England forced China to buy huge quotas of the narcotic at inflated prices, demonstrated the twin advantages of this gambit: easy money and addictive pacification. Today we have a double system. Both medical and criminal monopolies profiteer on various misery relievers. Heroin and cocaine long ago replaced overpriced gems as the best way for spies and death squads to raise extra cash. Synthetic endorphins made to mimic the brain's own contentment drugs, or perhaps analogues of pleasure-center neurotransmitters, might be promising assets for future speculation.

A black market also might develop for so-called PKCe pain relievers. Jon Levine and his coworkers at the Pain Center of the University of California at San Francisco have identified an enzyme, protein kinase C epsilon, which seems to be the transmitter used within pain-sensing neurons. If, as hoped, it is indeed a common denominator in most forms of pain from injury, the discovery could open the way for better, more universally effective analgesics. Like opioids, these might have highly attractive mental effects, as well as helping athletes play while injured and numbing a new generation of slam dancers.

In the next couple of decades, pharmacogenomics will give us hundreds of new drugs to modify consciousness. Many will be synthetic versions of natural substances. That's why the current campaign against gamma-hydroxybutyrate (GHB) is an especially ominous glimpse into the future.

GHB and its precursor molecule, gamma-butyrolacetone, are brain chemicals that increase the supply of gamma-aminobutyric acid (GABA), the "anti-anxiety neurotransmitter," which is also elevated by Valium and cannabis. Those who ingest GHB may fall suddenly into a deep sleep, and so it has sometimes been employed as a date-rape drug. Users taken to emergency rooms in "coma" by panic-stricken friends invariably awaken with no ill effects. Not a single report of fatal overdose has ever been substantiated, including the widely publicized death of River Phoenix in 1997. The actor died of a combined cocaine and heroin overdose. He had not used external GHB, but since GHB occurs naturally in the brain, it can *always* be found at autopsy. The news media and government press-release writers play up the scare for their own purposes, but they typically neglect to mention two actual dangers: toxic contaminants from amateur synthesis, now that it's illegal, and an interaction with alcohol that really *can* kill you.

Forty years of research have shown GHB supplements to be of value in alcohol and heroin withdrawal, childbirth, insomnia, workplace stress, and depressive states that include anxiety. In addition, it's less toxic than salt. Nevertheless, the Food and Drug Administration forced removal of GHB from the market in 1991 and is about to declare it medically useless, so the Drug Enforcement Agency can place it in Schedule I (the list of drugs whose users are to be persecuted most assiduously) along with heroin and marijuana.

This makes GHB the first naturally occurring component of the human brain to be outlawed. Almost certainly it will not be the last.

We're deciding some momentous questions on the drug battlefield. The war will determine whether choices of pleasure and pain relief are to be made by the person seeking them or by outside forces. Shall states of mind be held within narrow limits ordained from above and dispensed by a health-care industry that serves the corporate state? Or shall the individual be free to

modify his own consciousness at will? (So long as he doesn't endanger others—at the wheel, for example.)

And given the unavoidable truth that recreational medicine in
some form *will* exist, who shall profit from it? Small farmers?
Even—can we imagine such a thing?—no one? Or only big pharmas, doctors, lawyers, police, agency apparatchiks, organized
crime, and smugglers?

The sad truth is that, if Viagra grew on trees, it would be illegal. As a society, we're okay with drugs as long as the right dealer
gets paid.

Medicine in the Service of Tyranny

Medical techniques will soon enable others to reach inside one's
mind and twist the dials to their liking with a directness and accuracy never before possible. Even those who in the past have
dreamed of thought control through surreptitious mass drugging
never envisioned the methods aborning today.

Some of these techniques will immediately be put to work on
behalf of the drug warriors. For example, Kim Janda and his
coworkers at the Scripps Research Institute in California are testing a vaccine that they hope will cure a cocaine habit by causing
the immune system to deactivate the drug before it reaches the
brain. Xenova, a British biotech company, is testing a similar vaccine for cocaine, as well as one for nicotine.

A great advance in treatment, you may say—and medicine will
offer many such options in the future. Yet it remains to be seen
whether society's overseers will make them optionally available
or will force such vaccines against the currently prohibited drugs
upon students or job applicants, or everyone, without consent.

You may consider this a harmless, even benign development. But it doesn't take much imagination to extend the same techniques a little further. What if the antitobacco movement pushes nicotine all the way onto Schedule I? What if outrage over drunk driving combines with religious fundamentalism to bring back prohibition of alcohol? The scary truth is that this time it could be enforced: A vaccine spliced into the wheat in your pasta could make you throw up if you so much as have a glass of wine with your date.

Many other kinds of behavior-modifying drugs could be delivered through similar means. The technology already exists. Again, the initial applications seem benign. For example, a trial hepatitis B vaccine has been genetically engineered into potatoes. Other vaccines are planned for delivery via bananas, corn, tomatoes, soybeans, and other foods. Their potential for affordably protecting millions from certain diseases is very seductive. But food can be engineered to carry drugs as well as vaccines. Moreover, a vaccine can be made to immunize you against anything, even GHB or other chemicals normally found in your own body. Control of mind and mood, therapeutic or otherwise, could also be done with permanent living medicines—gut bacteria or human cells customized to secrete drugs or to jam this or that hormone.

Do we really want to let this technology loose? Inevitably it makes possible the paternalistic dosing of whole peoples against somebody's definition of bad traits, bad habits, bad feelings, or "antisocial tendencies" of thought caused by bad neurotransmitters.

Of course, the Dope War is a form of scapegoating. We've seen the pattern before. The majority blames its problems on a minority, whose faults are said to cause the problems that weigh everyone down. The cure is a purge—in genetic terms, removal of un-desirables from the breeding population. In twentieth-century Europe, Hitler and Stalin used the eugenics mumbo jumbo that their scientists provided to justify the genetic cleansing of about 20 million people. In the United States, a weaker eugenics move-ment led to the forced sterilization of 50,000 mental patients be-tween 1920 and 1972.

Tomorrow's upgrade medicine will widen the genetic differ-ences between and among populations. Now that we can all be made "normal," what are *you* doing out there on the fringe? How tempting for a law-and-order politician to offer "social harmony" or "violence prevention" by vaccine. The pitch will be even more seductive when made with an air of business efficiency and clini-cal detachment. Genetic medicine could be the perfect tool for new forms of social engineering.

The most dangerous of these efforts will be the ones that pro-ceed in secret. Intimate knowledge of brain chemistry will offer elites new ways to pursue psychological control of individual tar-gets and entire populations. This goal has lured American secret scientists for generations. In the mid-seventies, the Senate Select Committee on Intelligence, headed by Frank Church, a Demo-crat from Idaho, revealed dozens of mind-control experiments carried out on unwitting citizens in the fifties and sixties, includ-ing a notorious CIA program called MKULTRA, which involved surreptitiously dosing a subject with LSD, then subjecting him to hours of suggestion, manipulation, and interrogation. The Church committee also brought to light scores of CIA and Penta-gon contracts for other mind-control research, including work on methods of implanting posthypnotic suggestions uncon-sciously, even while the subject is asleep, using pulsed radio waves and microwaves.

The revelations surprised and disgusted many, but the committee never succeeded in getting details on current work, or even results and operational status of the techniques tested earlier. Without an American *glasnost* so we can know for sure, there is every reason to believe that such research has continued to this day and that some methods may be in use, abroad or even here. Some of the molecules discovered in the drug gold rush of the next decade are likely to induce docility, gullibility, and pliability better than any truth serum now known. They could be administered as easily as vaccines in Pablum.

Even if we in the First Nation of the First World tacitly ask our leaders to decimate the Third World so as to keep our privileges, do we really want them to enforce a Disneyfied blandness among ourselves, in the name of dysfunctional-family values or some such? On his 1930s *Mercury Theatre* radio program, Orson Welles did a play about a man who went to heaven. Eventually he grew bored with the eternal round of G-rated pastimes decreed by the Almighty. He asked permission to go to hell, only to be told, "You're *in* hell."

Whom Can We Trust with the Secrets of Life?

In April 1974, President Nixon and his national security adviser, Henry Kissinger, commissioned five agencies—the State Department, Central Intelligence Agency, Department of Defense, Department of Agriculture, and Agency for International Development—to produce a secret paper whose purpose was to forecast the effect of the Third World population explosion. National Security Study Memorandum 200 was delivered to President Ford in December 1974, and it became the guidebook for American foreign aid policy until it was declassified in 1989, presumably having been replaced by another secret memo.

The key finding presented in NSSM 200 was this: Less-developed countries (LDCs) with large land areas and diverse ecologies are potentially self-sufficient. Such nations will benefit in the short run from rapid population growth, which will increase their demographic and military clout relative to the much more slowly growing industrialized nations. Moreover, peoples with a high fertility rate have a younger average age than those with a low rate. That makes those LDCs more apt to demand economic independence from the Western multinationals, perhaps leading them to nationalize their own natural resources and thus jeopardize the flow of cheap oil and strategic metal ores. The report identified thirteen LDCs of special concern: India, Bangladesh, Pakistan, Nigeria, Mexico, Indonesia, Brazil, Thailand, the Philippines, Egypt, Turkey, Ethiopia, and Colombia.

Aside from the overall plan to exploit a genuine problem so as to maintain neocolonial economics, most of the rest of the memo is unobjectionable—simple good advice about helping to set up family-planning clinics, arranging better education and jobs for women, and so on. However, one paragraph briefly mentions an "alternate view," which holds that the Third World population problem is "less amenable to solution through voluntary measures than is generally accepted."

It would be hard to write a sentence more tantalizing to conspiracy researchers than that one. Nor is the subject all speculation. A parliamentary investigation in Brazil in 1991 found that millions of Brazilian women had been sterilized without their knowledge or consent in a program sponsored by the Agency for International Development.

People trying to piece together the extent of the U.S. "alternate" population program often refer to National Security Council Memo NSC–46, written in 1978 by Kissinger's successor, Zbigniew Brzezinski, and revealed via the Freedom of Information Act. In it Brzezinski recommends using FBI and CIA "special clandestine operations" to sow dissension among black leaders in the United States and Africa, especially to prevent cooperation between them, and to collect "sensitive information" on black UN representatives opposed to our apartheid-era African policies. The memo does not mention population control, but no great mental leap is required to imagine it in a related memo yet to be uncovered. Evidence of continued strategic importance given to the subject comes from an early-1980s CIA paper called "Population, Resources, and Politics in the Third World: The Long View." This report also was pried loose via the Freedom of Information Act, but the parts dealing specifically with methods of population control had been deleted.

What tools will genetic technology offer such people in the future? The *documented* budget for secret projects by the CIA alone now exceeds $30 billion a year. We can expect the post-9/11 war on terrorism to increase the budget and decrease the restraints on its use. Leaving aside the consequences for democracy, what medical consequences would result—are resulting?—from biogenocide by a regime able to keep its actions secret?

Americans like to believe that their "bad old days" of genocide, slavery, apartheid, and imperialism are safely in the past, or at least safely overseas. But millions of U.S. citizens and countless others around the world know enough recent history to distrust the political, military, and business factions that control our government and our other leading institutions. And it's clear that these are the very factions that will exert a dominating influence over the shape and purposes of biotech medicine. It's also clear that this medical research will yield weapons that will give new meaning to the term "live ordnance." They could be used to wield unprecedented control over individuals, over populations, and over life itself.

The emergence of molecular control technologies raises a truly Darwinian question of survival for much of the human race. Perhaps Americans can plan safe and worthy use of biotech medicine only after we confront our true place in the world and learn to see ourselves as others see us. Until then, trusting our secret agencies with the keys to life could be the worst policy decision since Montezuma showed Cortés the Gold Room.

PART THREE

Alternative Futures

CHAPTER 12

Medicine
in the Balance

AS FAR AS CRITIQUES OF CAPITALISM are concerned, a great hush has fallen over the earth since the demise of Soviet communism. But perhaps the psychedelic shaman and anthropologist Terence McKenna was prescient. In the early nineties he optimistically quipped, "Communism was just the *first* to go."

In its heyday, the Soviet military machine consumed an astounding 30 to 40 percent of the USSR's gross domestic product. Its lust for resources in an economy much smaller than ours was the greatest single factor in communism's collapse. With the subsequent decline of the ruble and the downsizing of Russia's armed forces, the American medical machine has now become the largest economic entity on earth. It's also the one with the greatest potential for straining our global economic system to the breaking point.

The American Nonsystem

With the single glaring exception of the former Soviet empire, all other industrialized nations have approximately the same level of medical technology as the United States, yet they keep health-care costs under a tenth of GDP–on average, about half the U.S. level. In each case the elements of success are the same. They consist of one *what* and three *hows*. The *what* is a preference for simple medicine, which is enforced by the *hows*, which together constitute a system for making health care serve society instead of vice versa.

The art of healing with herbs and other natural remedies, broadly termed holistic medicine or naturopathy, might be called the people's medicine. Its beginnings go back at least sixty thousand years. Here and there throughout the world, study continues on genetically unmodified plants, unpatentable herbs that have yielded, among recent examples, clinically proven mixtures for osteoarthritis and prostatitis. In terms of research capital and prestige, however, holistic medicine is very much the poor cousin of stainless-steel allopathy, which is paradoxically labeled both "modern" and "traditional" medicine.

Even so, naturopathy is gaining some ground in the United States, causing fears about loss of market share among drug vendors. In 1994, a public outcry induced Congress, behind the leadership of Senator Orrin Hatch of Utah, a Republican, to pass the Dietary Supplement Health and Education Act. This law forced the Food and Drug Administration to back off from a plan to remove nature's remedies from the realm of popular choice. The FDA had intended to classify most vitamins, minerals, herbs, and nutrient extracts as prescription drugs. Similar pressure later led the agency to recognize the legitimacy of acupuncture, and then to allow advertising of supplements to treat "natural conditions"–common ailments called by their popular names.

A gradually increasing number of Americans use natural methods for prevention, as a first resort for minor problems, and as an alternative or adjunct treatment of serious illness. Some M.D.s now incorporate holistic medicine's accumulated wisdom into their practices. By heading off trouble before it gets serious, naturopathy slows the rise in medical costs somewhat.

Other nations spend less than we do on health care in part because they emphasize the low-tech approach in a much more systematic and widespread way. It's built into their systems instead of being considered an oddball relic for individual doctors and patients to seek out on their own.

Foreign arrangements also save money by these common denominators of structure, the three *hows* mentioned above.

1. A centralized, state-run, tax-funded payment system operates under one set of rules for everybody. This eliminates secrecy, much of the administrative waste, and most of the opportunities for fraud that are endemic to our overly complex, private-public hybrid–our "nonsystem."

2. State control of spending usually imposes delays and bureaucratic hurdles for *elective* treatments, even for the well-off. Savings are a result.

3. Universal or near-universal coverage and reasonably efficient service for *therapeutic* medicine make for general public confidence in the system. Perceived fairness not only frees society from the expensive consequences of leaving the poor without health care (discussed below). It also helps to defuse class hatreds.

The result is a health-care system most citizens are basically satisfied with. Polls show that no other industrial nation's people would trade their setup for ours.

Some say that other countries spend less than we do because they reap the fruits of research done in the United States. There's some truth to that argument. However, it ignores the fact that most industrialized nations support vigorous research efforts, both public and private, while considering our developmental frenzy excessive, in that it takes money away from proven ways of promoting health.

It's also claimed that cost controls in Eurasia create shortfalls that prompt international companies to jack up American prices to subsidize the use of drugs and other health-care products overseas. Again, the argument turns on excess. If a nation's cost mandates didn't include a profit margin, companies would simply stop doing business there. The fact that they don't only highlights the degree of profiteering that exists in America's revved-up market.

In any case, no study has ever found either of these factors significant compared to the overall structure of national health plans abroad.

By contrast, the nonsystem by which health care is managed in the United States seems designed to encourage swindles, increase class animosity, and favor the rich over the sick. These costs amount to an exorbitant social and financial burden that all Americans help to carry. Are we reenacting in health care the 1920s–1930s scenario of unrestrained speculation, financial collapse, revolt, counterrevolt, and legislative intervention that almost destroyed the world financial system? If so, we may be halfway through a fascinating and scary socioeconomic experiment.

Victor Fuchs, a professor of economics at Stanford and a longtime critic of American medicine, has said that there may come a time when health-care reform will be the *easy* way out. He may be right.

Three Roads to the Future

If someday we want to think seriously about subjugating medicine to the needs of society, there are basically three roads we can take.

First, we can decide not to. We'll create a completely laissez-faire setup. Let health care be a Wild West saloon brawl, everyone fending for him- or herself in a pure-retail system. Health care will be an unregulated form of merchandise. It will probably still be somewhat controlled for quality, but its availability will be entirely a matter of personal wealth. The health-care industry will offer a range of value, from the secondhand Yugo to the customized Ferrari Testarossa. It'll be accepted that a large number of Americans will have no wheels at all.

For those who can afford to drive, the business will be relatively efficient, based on a direct relationship between buyer and seller. The only restraints will be those of the market (which favors better merchandise when it has an informed choice), plus whatever safeguards consumer advocates and government watchdogs can provide.

Alternatively, we can ask government to level the playing field, à la Scandinavia. Health care will be a right of citizenship, standardized at an adequate level–the serviceable family sedan. In return for this security, we'll all share more or less equally a high rate of taxes. We'll trade the inefficiencies of the market for those of a reasonably fair state bureaucracy.

This second road would obviously require a top-to-bottom overhaul of the current medical payment system by legislative fiat–over the dead bodies of the insurance industry, the HMO industry, the hospital industry, the biotechnology and pharmaceutical industries, and the advertising industry. Such a radical change sounds impossible in the United States right now, but given a few well-timed scandals, an accumulation of blatant injustices, and a handful of startling disasters produced by genetic engineering or other new-medicine technologies, it might become less inconceivable. Honest physicians, nurses, and other health-care workers–the vast majority–would be natural allies of the general public in the struggle.

Of course, even this kind of revolution won't solve all our medical problems. Capitalized medicine has its strengths, especially speed and prolificacy–the pace of discovery and the profusion of products, at least in some stages of the market's evolution.

Wealth will always have advantages, of course. And demands for equal access to health care, instead of being satisfied or denied by the marketplace, would be fought in the legislature as each new wave of treatments breaks. Nor would state control eliminate fraud altogether. A few clever souls will hack into any payment scheme we might devise. All we can do is decrease the openings for fraud by making the system fair and simple.

There is a third possible road: We can—and most likely we will—jury-rig a hybrid combining some of the pros and cons of each of the first two models. In other words, we can continue to work within our current nonsystem, tinkering around the edges.

In the foreseeable future, the momentum and emphasis increasingly will go toward the laissez-faire road, but we are not likely to get rid of public medical assistance entirely. In the American health-care system of the next generation, a basic, often inadequate level of therapeutic care will remain a right for some, provided by a "physician underclass" who cling to their altruism despite ever-declining incomes.

For those at the other end of the economic scale, medicine will be an infinitely upgradable commodity, leading to the new heaven of genetic rejuvenation. And for those in between, it will be affordable or not, depending on one's job, income, and luck. In the middle and lower economic classes, moreover, basic therapeutic family medicine will be marginalized, starved for cash and talent, while money rains down on the glamorous genetic-enhancement fields.

We can expect many to go without health care almost entirely, especially the one sixth of the population (about 45 million Americans) who have no insurance. That proportion is rising rapidly and seems to keep pace with the percentage of GDP we devote to medicine, also about one sixth. We can expect that as medical spending grows, this group will also grow to a fourth or third of the citizenry.

The rising number of uninsured is economically significant in part because these people are not entirely outside the system. They go without care until they have a health crisis. Then they visit a publicly subsidized emergency room or clinic, where medicine plays catch-up, operating in its least efficient and most expensive mode.

Many cities tried to save money in the mid-nineties by closing their public hospitals or selling them to the big for-profit chains. Often they saw their savings evaporate as the poor, delayed by new hurdles yet mandated some sort of care somewhere, by Medicaid or the state constitution, finally showed up in the back wards of the private hospitals, sicker than ever. Hence any expected savings from exclusion actually hide a net loss to society, even without counting the costs in human suffering and lost productivity. As noted above, under our current system that net loss grows disproportionately the more we all spend on medicine.

A Right or a Privilege—Who Decides?

There's that nagging question again: Is health care a right, or is it a privilege, a commodity to be bought and sold for whatever price the market will bear?

In terms of *who* gets covered, Americans have already decided that health care is fundamentally a commodity, for sale at a profit. There's little chance of a new debate over a national health plan, at least not until costs hurt a lot more than they do now.

There's a "boiled frog" quality to the escalation of costs. We get used to a burden that would've been intolerable a generation ago, the way a frog supposedly doesn't notice it's being cooked if the temperature of the water rises slowly enough. Vast improvements in medical technique make us avid for more, willing to overlook the cumulative cost. To cite one typical example, cataract and gallbladder removal, which 20 years ago were failure-prone surgeries needing long hospital stays, have become hour-long outpatient procedures of astonishing safety and benefit. Now upgrade medicine will change the terms, and the rights question will be argued in a million skirmishes over *what* gets covered.

Should all improvements be considered health care and thus be covered by existing plans—full speed ahead and damn the premiums? What lines, if any, shall we draw? Should my employer's plan cover a baldness treatment that makes me more confident and thus better at my job (but also more likely to seek a better one)? Should my taxes and premiums help pay for your waistline-improvement therapy? Does the answer change if I might fall in love with you as a result of it? Should a genetic upgrade to my mathematical skills be deductible on my income-tax form? For that matter, if genetic improvements are reimbursable, do corporate retreats, New Age workshops, and meditation classes now fit under the rubric of medicine? Or do we want a retrenchment, so that insurance covers only drugs and technology that are therapeutic in the strictest sense?

Answers to questions like these are easy to formulate in the abstract, but when your interests, or mine, are directly involved, the issues become much harder.

We've already foreseen the outlines of this struggle in the year of Viagra. It was originally approved by the FDA in 1998 for use by a moderately large market—men with clinically assessed erectile dysfunction. But doctors have the legally assured freedom to prescribe a drug for a patient who does not have the indicated condition, as long as the doctor believes that the drug will help the person.

As a result, a large proportion, perhaps as high as 90 percent, of Viagra prescriptions are "recreational." Because Medicaid must pay benefits for all approved medical treatments, suddenly the federal government became the all-time biggest promoter of the sex lives of poor people. Laws being inconsistent, Medicare did not cover the drug, putting the government in the position of saying, "Over sixty-five? We think you're too old for Viagra." Private insurers and workplace plans varied widely in their Viagra policies. Some said yes, meaning, "Sex is a part of healthy life." Some said no, meaning, "Sex is a luxury." And some limited coverage to, say, six pills a month—in effect deciding what frequency turns intercourse from a necessity into a luxury.

Those who establish national health-care policies face similar issues. Britain's National Health Service decided not to cover Viagra. Its directors publicly worried that it might crowd out more life-critical treatments and privately feared the cost, estimated to be as much as $1.7 billion per year. Poland, on the other hand, troubled by a steeply declining birth rate, has cut contraception subsidies in favor of funds for Viagra.

Sometimes the decision-making has unexpected benefits. In Japan, aging senior managers of the Ministry of Health and Welfare got Viagra approved for use in Japan in six months, though an application for a low-dose birth control pill had languished in the ministry for ten years (the ministry is staffed—coincidentally?—by 198 men and only six women). The real reasons may have had more to do with abortionists' and condom makers' fear of competition from the birth control pill, but in any case the injustice became laughably clear, and the pill finally came to Japan in July 1999, three months after Viagra.

On this side of the Pacific, demand by upper-middle-class men for Viagra payments created a fairness backlash that resulted in a mandate to finally get coverage of contraception by most states, by women's prescription plans, and by the Federal Equal Opportunity Employment Commission. After all, with the Defense Department paying $50 million a year to raise morale with Viagra, the inequity had become indefensible. But not embarrassing, it seems. In April 2001, the administration of George Bush the younger removed coverage for contraception from federal workers' insurance.

The answer to each reimbursement question depends on who asks it. "What is the proper scope of my responsibility for you?" sounds different from "What is the proper scope of your responsibility for me?" For you, "growing old gracefully" means accepting your decline without making my insurance rates go up. For me, it means having the body of a 20-something until I die in my sleep at the age of 100. (Make that 200.)

Some analysts are hinting that insurers may adjust coverage on the basis of a client's economic status, using such measures as projected lifetime earnings and "value to society" (translation: total expected premiums). Now you can see why *my* collagen injections are more essential than *your* prosthesis.

Consider the amazing surgical techniques that promise correction of spina bifida in the womb, soon to be applied as well to hydrocephaly and other congenital abnormalities. Nothing could be more medically necessary for the well-being of the infant. Most parents can be expected to lay down their last dollar for it, if need be. And yet, is it right to make the collective pay, or even to let the parents pay, to save the lives of infants who otherwise would die soon after birth, while so many healthy children languish for want of adoptive parents?

There will be thousands of medical advances in the coming decades, and almost every one will force us to go through the same agonizing calibrations of fairness–unless and until we by consensus form a coherent national policy for deciding what shall be paid by society, what by risk pools, and what left to the individual.

Is Insurance in the Cards?

All the questions of fairness are going to be further complicated by changes that genetic technology may force in our nonsystem of medical payment.

Shared risk is the fundamental economic and social concept behind insurance. If insurers now begin to tailor contracts closely to individuals based on their *personal* risk profiles, they may end up undermining the rationale for buying insurance in the first place.

Today every medical purchase is centrally indexed, as anyone who has filled a prescription for Viagra or Celebrex knows from the number of direct-mail solicitations he soon receives for other sex or arthritis products. All that data will make it easier for underwriters to draft policies only for the problems a customer is least likely to have, or to set extremely profitable rates for genuine coverage.

You already know the power ratio between the typical insurance company and the typical insurance customer: "Please take a moment to review these documents. If you have any questions, skip lunch to dial 1-800-YOU-LOSE when all representatives are currently assisting other customers. Your call is very important to us. Please stay on the line and have the last four digits of your next of kin ready." To redress that balance of power just a little, we suggest one simple clause to be required in every policy, backed by accounting guidelines checkable by state insurance regulators: "Approximately x cents of the average premium dollar under this contract will be paid out in benefits."

Yet at their moment of greatest triumph, genetic screening and UHI cards might wipe out insurance companies altogether. The ability to predict and preempt disease would knock the whole notion of risk sharing into a cocked hat. When risk is known with certainty, there is in effect no risk, only anticipated future health-care expenses that people can plan for on their own without paying underwriters.

The Internet will make it easier to match such planning products to the market. There will be online medical malls, letting people build their own health plan from prefab modules. That approach will isolate the individual and preclude volume discounts. There is an alternative, however: A company (now defunct) called Mercata.com pioneered the idea of an online group buying service based on medical affinity groups. Current and future diabetics, asthmatics, and so on will band together for tailored coverage from risk-factor management programs—in effect, one-disease HMOs. Instead of what professionals think people need, the criterion will become what people know they want. That spells trouble for the person predisposed to heart disease who unexpectedly gets cancer, but then, full-body medical armor is part of the incentive for getting rich.

Oddly enough, losing the insurers may not cut society's medical bill. Preventive intervention will dramatically reduce treatment costs for some diseases, to be sure, but the total number of available services will grow exponentially. Since medicine will be able to do much more, per capita buying will rise, slowly in defined-contribution (fixed-spending) employee plans and rapidly in the wealthier classes.

In addition, most of the advances forecast for the new era of medicine are in the area of drugs, broadly defined—including traditional pharmaceuticals, gene activators and inhibitors, gene-replacement therapies, and implants of hormone-delivering contraptions or cells. Moreover, many of them will entail lifelong or recurrent maintenance. In fact, the market gives drug companies a tremendous incentive to avoid one-shot cures in favor of products for long-term treatment.

Compared with years past, then, an ever-increasing percentage of medicine's options and expenses will flow from and to the pharmas, whose revenue streams are already overflowing. Now that we have exhausted our supply-side cost-control options, like managed care, the drug flood will make employers run screaming to exit health care altogether, despite the move to defined contributions. And the 2000 election stalemate foretells no help from Washington.

So, along with balancing the checkbook and managing the portfolio, every responsible upwardly mobilized adult will learn to allocate income for predicted lifetime health-care needs. As the complexity of shopping choices grows, a new layer of medical middlemen and infobrokers will replace insurers. The banking and debt industries will design new services to profit from helping the individual develop her strategy. An explosive increase in choices among competing products for prevention and enhancement will accelerate the shift to retail among all but the very poor. Convenience, brand names, designer surgery, and celebrity-spokesmodeled body and mind upgrades will be far more heavily promoted than today. All these factors combined will make the health-care insurance system unsustainable.

Then, at some point—between 2010 and 2020?—a repugnant level of class stratification, along with middle-class pressure for greater access, may create the political conditions needed to reform medicine in part as a public utility. There could be a tax-subsidized fix for some of the worst inequities, further increasing total costs. A genetic New Deal might be forthcoming to forestall both revolt and complete equality. It's a truism among health-policy mavens that America really wants to switch back and forth every ten years between private ownership and public stewardship. The new gene-based medicine might create such an oscillating health-care engine.

As Costs Keep Rising

Optimists predict huge savings from the new medical interventions. For example, they posit genetically based cures for heart disease and cancer, then subtract current costs for these illnesses, roughly one fourth of all medical spending. However, such a picture ignores the likely gradual and difficult progress through the complexities of multigene interactions in these diseases, as well as the initially high cost of treatments, each of which must be priced to recoup development costs and earn profits before something better comes along.

For example, Schering-Plough recently combined its old antiviral drug ribavirin with its lab-grown interferon alfa–2b, one of the first commercial products of biotech medicine. The pairing, called Rebetron, is twice as effective as either drug alone against hepatitis C, the slow virus that kills some 10,000 Americans a year from liver damage. Since hepatitis C produces $600 million a year in medical costs, not counting liver transplants, we might be tempted to credit that amount to savings a few years hence.

But wait. Rebetron clears the virus in only about one third of patients, and about one fourth of those suffer a relapse. Each 48-week course of treatment costs $17,000. Researchers think they can predict which one in three the drug will help. One third of the 4 million Americans infected with hepatitis C equals 1.3 million people, or a potential market of about $20 billion. If half of these people were to buy the treatment over the next five years, that would more than triple our costs for hepatitis C. Moreover, it is reasonable to expect a better treatment to arrive in five years, which would still have a market twice as large as Rebetron's (the two thirds of patients whom Rebetron fails to help), even without new cases.

The rosy predictions of savings also ignore the vast new market for elective upgrades, as well as longer life spans in which to purchase them. How exactly will we hold down medical expenses when we're running to the doctor for the latest brainware? It's a fundamental law of capitalism: No profitable market goes unexploited. Nor will governmental restraints, even if they could be enacted, help much. The corollary is this: If a market cannot be exploited legally, it will be exploited illegally—at much higher cost to the individual and to society.

Most important, such Pollyanna predictions assume that the genetic revolution will consist entirely of miracles. They ignore the inevitable downside of any new technology—the hidden obstacles, the unforeseen social effects of even beneficent changes, the cost of accidents, and the potential for misuse.

However, if we focus only on the miracles and their costs, monetary and otherwise, we will have missed the point. Further upstream there is a principle involved that is more fundamental than deciding who gets how much coverage for what. We use the phrase "the best justice money can buy" to express our cynicism about lawyers and courts. Behind the sarcasm, though, we still maintain our ideal of a system blind to all outside influences. Yet we refer to "the best medical care money can buy" without a trace of irony. Shouldn't we—didn't we, not so long ago—expect the same degree of impartiality from medicine?

How Smart Choices Can Help: The Orphan Drug Act

To sum up, then, any attempt to reform medicine faces a challenge that is at least fourfold. It must:

1. Save money by restoring the balance between high- and low-technology health care
2. Do so without halting medical progress
3. Reconcile competing needs in apportioning coverage
4. Restore some level of equality and universal access to health care

In trying to fit medicine with justice's blindfold, we can draw upon at least one positive experience that shows how smart lawmaking can benefit everyone and make health-care delivery more equitable—the Orphan Drug Law of 1983.

One of nature's greatest challenges to modern medicine is the group of diseases collectively called "orphans." These are some five thousand illnesses, most of them debilitating and fatal, each of which individually strikes too few people to attract the funding needed to find cures or treatments. All together, though, they afflict about 20 million Americans.

To help solve this funding problem, in 1981 the California congressman Henry Waxman—who is also a physician—proposed the Orphan Drug Act, which became law at the beginning of 1983. Waxman sought to give drug companies financial incentives to find cures. Chief among these are tax credits for research and the right to market any effective drug exclusively for seven years—essentially an extension of patent protection to substances that might not otherwise be patentable. The law included a means test to determine which diseases should be considered orphans and how much tax credit to extend against the manufacturer's potential profit from the market.

Before 1983, only about a dozen drugs had been developed for such low-frequency illnesses. Since then, some 220 have been introduced, with another 800 in testing. Pulmozyme (dornase alpha) and TOBI (tobramycin) help prevent lung damage from cystic fibrosis, enabling many CF patients to live into their forties and fifties instead of dying in their teens. Remicade (infliximab) reduces the severe bowel inflammation of Crohn's disease. Droxia (hydroxyurea), an obsolete cancer chemotherapy drug, helps against sickle-cell anemia. Ontak (denileukin diftitox) sometimes controls a rare cancer, cutaneous T-cell lymphoma. Mepron (atovaquone) is the first effective drug against pneumocystic pneumonia, a lung infection often fatal to AIDS patients. The value of thalidomide in Hansen's disease (leprosy) was discovered under the law's provisions. The list is long and steadily growing.

By common consent, the Orphan Drug Act is one of the best laws ever passed, an example of legislation done right. Aspects of it have been copied by Japan, Australia, Canada, Sweden, France, and the United Kingdom. A version is under study by the European Union.

Nonetheless, its interaction with for-profit medicine leaves room for improvement. For one thing, although its exclusive-marketing provision makes it easier to test old drugs and natural substances for rare diseases, that only points up the fact that similar research on more common ailments is neglected by comparison.

For another thing, the law has made rare diseases *too* profitable, some say. When the bill was first passed, the pharmas thought the deal wasn't sweet enough and showed little interest in it. Therefore Congress amended the law, allowing even patentable drugs to qualify for orphan financial benefits. Moreover, Congress eliminated the means test, instead simply defining orphan diseases as those that afflict no more than 200,000 Americans. This allowed drug companies to define subsets of *any* disease as an orphan to get the law's benefits, a process known in the trade as "salami slicing." For example, similar cancers in different organs may be considered distinct illnesses in terms of the law.

Even when used legitimately, the amended law has generated handsome revenues, though not always reasonable access to treatment. Since about four fifths of the genuine orphan diseases are caused by single-gene defects, the Orphan Drug Act has been and will continue to be a prime mover in the early development of genetic medicine. So far, as a group orphan drugs have been by far biotech's most profitable sector.

An AIDS patient's annual bill for Glaxo-Wellcome's Retrovir (AZT, zidovudine) begins at $10,000, and as of the late nineties the drug had brought the company well over $3 billion in sales. Genzyme's Ceredase (alglucerase) is used to treat Gaucher's disease, a syndrome of anemia, dementia, and fragile bones caused by defective cellular metabolism of fats. Ceredase was discovered, developed, and tested with public money from the National Institutes of Health, but since 1991 it has generated an average of $150 million a year in private revenue for Genzyme. Other examples of blockbuster profits from orphans include Genentech's Protropin (human growth hormone) and Amgen's Epogen (recombinant human erythropoietin), which is used to treat various types of anemia.

Of course, profits in themselves are not evil. But profiteering on top of high per-dose costs of manufacture means *very* high prices. Ceredase treatment for Gaucher's disease runs $100,000 to $600,000 a year. Since we lack any semblance of universal insurance coverage, especially for drugs–some two thirds of drug expenses are paid for out of pocket–many orphan-disease sufferers can see their medicines way up on the top shelf but can't reach that high.

Various new amendments to the law have been proposed, such as shortening the exclusive marketing period, assessing royalties for use of publicly funded research that leads to an orphan drug, or requiring payback of tax credits above a certain profit level, which would go into subsidized purchases of the drugs. Given the extraordinarily high revenues per patient, however, such ploys are unlikely to make much of a dent in prices. Besides, drug company lobbying power makes a return to the stricter provisions of the original Waxman bill unlikely. Perhaps only the unthinkable–price controls and a national health policy–can help.

Such considerations bring up, as always, questions of fairness in allocation. Batches of some drugs are limited in size by investment constraints, so that even among patients able to pay, the recipients must be chosen by lottery or date of application. Is a new subsidy in order here?

Finally, most orphan diseases remain orphans, with no cure in sight. Hunter's syndrome, a cluster of problems stemming from defective heart valves, which dooms its sufferers to painful lives and early deaths, still has no treatment, even though its causative gene defect was discovered more than a decade ago. Should the government step in to subsidize a research push for this disease? If so, for how many others?

Certain more widespread hereditary diseases, such as cystic fibrosis, the most common hereditary disease of whites, and sickle cell anemia, the most common in blacks, are "crossovers," with large enough markets to attract some private investment. Should orphan drug support be scaled back for them? Do we want tiers on the basis of the incidence of various diseases, with such illnesses as multiple sclerosis, amyotrophic lateral sclerosis (Lou Gehrig's disease), muscular dystrophy, and total (gray-only) color blindness on the next level down? For that matter, are we ready for a more global view? Is it more important to treat 16,000 new cases of nonfatal Lyme disease among suburban Americans each year, or to deal with a million deaths from malaria among the foreign poor?

In a few years, a standard way to overwrite faulty DNA with genetic Ko-Rec-Type may make these questions easier by lowering the cost of many therapies, both orphan and non-orphan. Unless and until that happens, the early rewards of biotech medicine will likely bypass many of those whom we once assumed it would benefit first.

How Far Should We Go?

Most orphan diseases are caused by single-gene defects. Doctors in the future presumably will try to cure them with genetic therapy rather than alleviate them with the kinds of drugs available today. Yet developers of genetic therapies for these rare diseases will face the same financial obstacles as orphan drug designers. The question of how we as a society will respond to this "orphan gene" problem is important—and not only for the lives involved (as if that weren't enough). It's also an early example of the long series of questions that genetic medicine will raise. And, up to a point, it's one of the easy ones. Either we care about the less fortunate and find a way to help them or we don't. Moreover, anyone can be on the wrong side of the dilemma. Since every one of us has *something* wrong in our genes, and since, as pharmacogenomics teaches, each of us has a unique pattern of susceptibilities, we're all potential orphans.

After we've sorted out all the sticky questions of social duty, rights, and policy, we still won't be done. We'll be up against another moral question, the hardest kind, one with no possible "right" answer, only a delicate balance in the gray area: How far do we want to go in treating genetic diseases?

Enabling people with genetic ailments to live long, happy lives will increase the frequency of the typos in the genetic library. Is that just a price we'll gladly pay for helping people in the present? Of course we realize, hiding a guilty smile, that it will guarantee markets for the future. On the other hand, do we really want to embark on the course of large-scale germ-line therapy, genetically engineering future generations in an effort to eliminate every defect once and for all? That means being sure the de-

248

fects have no hidden purpose and trusting technicians to spell-check our code without introducing worse bugs.

No enormous enterprise like genetic medicine can be all good or all evil. Throughout most of this book, we've been looking at medical problems that result from human nature. But the underlying suffering is much too real, and the cry for relief is also part of human nature. Let our exasperation with the flaws of capitalized medicine not obscure the challenges we face from *in*human nature.

Consider this example: Since 1993, geneticists have learned the cause of the progressive and fatal dementia called Huntington's chorea, the disease that killed the folksinger Woodie Guthrie. It's a kind of genetic stutter. Within nerve cells there is a certain protein, now called huntingtin. Except for the ends, it consists of a long stretch of glutamine molecules. Sometimes, while reading the code for this long string, the transcription enzymes lose their place, slip backward, and insert extra glutamines. Each time the brain cell divides thereafter, the repetitions are likely to double and redouble. The protein becomes an unusable mess that clogs up the cells so they can no longer function.

Today the number of superfluous repeats can be counted to tell the unlucky carrier, with accuracy to within a year or two, when he will lose his mind and die. But there is as yet no treatment.

Here's another example of imperfect nature's careless cruelty: Some people have a variant of a certain gene called p56Ick. When these people are infected with the coxsackie virus, one of the most common of those that cause the common cold, their immune systems begin to destroy the muscle cells of their hearts. Josef Penninger and others at the Amgen Institute, in Toronto, and at the Ontario Cancer Center of the University of Toronto have recently shown that this interaction is the chief cause of heart attacks in young people, and probably in many older people as well.

The more extreme critics of genetic medicine often portray its practitioners as so many Dr. Frankensteins eager to loose their monsters upon a warm and cuddly Gaia. We, too, worry about the overeager pursuit of genetic powers and their heedless application in the quest for profit. But nature can also be monstrous in its arbitrary cruelty. In the real world, the Big It—nature, God, the Great Mother, Allah, the Tao, Pan, the quantum void, the universe—is as indifferent to the health of the individual as a falling rock. Compassion for human beings comes from human beings. Or not. It's that simple.

And yet . . .

There is a balance that must assert itself, or we may be putting ourselves in ultimate danger. With language, our marvelous ability to bequeath life's lessons to our descendants across the boundary of death, we humans have hauled ourselves almost completely out of the food chain. So successful have we been that we eat other animals by the billions and exterminate any that still occasionally presume to eat one of us. Except for those we adopt as pets, we treat other creatures as things, because we cannot imagine ourselves as nourishment. We even keep our dead in sterile cocoons lest via bacteria and worms they should rejoin the web of being.

Now we plan to take our industrialization of animals a step further, reducing them to living vats whom we will force to grow whatever we desire by means of bizarre, debilitating mutations. Our quest for medical omnipotence through genetics will inevitably reinforce our tendency to think, in our immature arrogance, that we are better than life—"too cool for the room." If we pay no heed to the cautionary voices among us, sooner or later life may let us know we're still part of it by taking a big bite. Even should we master the earth without catastrophe, as we reach the stars we will find ourselves once again junior members, part of a larger ecology that may rudely shake our upstart pride.

Nature is tricky. Examples of the dangers that arise when we ignore this truth are numerous. Two of them are related to one of medicine's greatest triumphs—the conquest of polio.

One recent theory on the origin of AIDS suggests that it jumped to humans via tests on Africans of batches of the Sabin oral polio vaccine that were contaminated with residual chimpanzee kidney tissue from its preparation. (However, a recent review of the evidence presented to the Royal Society of London cast doubt on this idea.)

The breakthrough weapon against polio, the Salk vaccine, was administered to 98 million Americans between 1955 and 1963. It has long been known to have contained SV40, a simian virus from the monkey kidney tissue in which it was prepared. In the early 1960s, several studies seemed to have proved the virus harmless to humans, even though, as Beatrice Eddy had shown, it readily causes cancer in other animals. Indeed, it became a standard lab tool, since one of its constituents is the most oncogenic (cancer-producing) protein ever discovered. Now recent work has implicated the virus as at least a cofactor in mesothelioma, a rare, fast-growing, and almost uniformly fatal cancer of the chest wall that was previously thought to be triggered only by exposure to asbestos. Mesothelioma was all but unknown before the polio vaccine. The SV40 virus may also be the sole cause of several deadly, long-onset brain and bone cancers.

If either or both of these theories turn out to be true, then the conquest of polio, one of the proudest achievements in all of medicine, could end up costing more lives than it saved. There may be times when we have no choice but to "take our deads," as boys of an earlier generation used to put it when we played at cowboys and Indians. Lying down in pretend death for a few minutes when we got "shot" was essential to keep the game honest.

What does it all prove? That the war against polio was in vain? That humans have no business tampering with the arbitrary plans of nature? Surely not. Our minds and talents are part of the natural order, too, and we probably couldn't stop using them even if we tried. But in the face of all we don't understand, a certain restraint is in order, an awareness that there will always be an imperfect match between human aspirations and the unknowable demands of nature.

The Ends
of Medicine

WE'VE USED A LOT OF QUESTION
marks in this book. Not only is the future hard to predict, but also we are trying to forecast the outcome of advances
in medicine, a development that in
some ways is a curse and in some ways
is one of our greatest blessings.

There's an analogy in the sickle cell
anemia gene. When passed on to a child
by both parents, it creates the disease.
When bequeathed by only one, it gives

resistance to malaria. Socially, we're groping for a way to enjoy the benefits of medicine without getting sick from a double dose.

We meet that pro-and-con dichotomy throughout our health-care system. The conversion of medicine into a profit-seeking industry forces it to give short shrift to health and to focus on expensive technological cures—which nonetheless will work many wonders heretofore impossible. New openness to sexual therapies improves millions of lives but causes large new expenditures. Nowhere are goods and evils so intertwined, or so crucial to separate, as in the medicine of the future.

The Biggest Questions

Ethical questions concerning genetic science have received, to put it kindly, sporadic public discussion. Debates over safeguards in recombinant DNA research were widely aired during the 1970s, and the two-year moratorium on research that emerged from the National Academy of Science's Conference on Recombinant DNA, commonly called the Asilomar Conference, showed that pure science can respond with restraint. But in the 1980s and early 1990s, several court decisions that allowed life forms to be patented and thus set the course of the entire biotechnology industry passed by with scarcely a flicker on the view-screen of public attention. Control of that industry should have been a central issue of the 2000 election, but it was never even on the agenda.

We are entering a new era of medicine from which we have every reason to expect a great deal. Yet public discourse on the issues has tended to focus on just a few of them. For example, there has been much debate over the source of embryonic research tissue, over the rights and wrongs of human cloning, and over the future ability of parents to customize their children.

Relatively little attention has been paid to numerous matters that are far more pressing. What about the ethics of genetic ownership and compensation, especially as embodied in the worldwide recolonization of the weak by the strong? What about medicalizing more and more aspects of human life at the expense of personal initiative and control? How will biotechnological enhancements, many conferring godlike powers and being too pricey for all but a few, affect our increasingly divergent economic classes? How will these new powers interact with certain contradictions in our social system, such as that between the commercialized cult of individualism versus the urge to control other people's behavior, as embodied in laws against victimless crimes; or the conflict between free enterprise and the incessant working of official conspiracies against the general good, as typified by "Vitamins Incorporated," the great global vitamin scam, and the use of unwitting people as test subjects?

Today we stand poised for a genomics-based revolution, which, along with other advances in medicine, results from accelerated public- and private-sector investment. At the same time, we are beset by grave doubts about how to manage our explosively growing health-care system, as its thirst for resources seems unquenchable. Those who set public policy will have to answer—or culpably ignore—at least four overriding questions:

1. How can breakthrough therapeutic benefits be distributed fairly through an overloaded, largely private, and increasingly proprietary health-care-delivery system that is generally recognized to be an abject failure in terms of efficiency, equity, and rationality?

2. A large and increasing portion of medicine will be nontherapeutic, designed to improve normal human capacities and lifestyles, not cure disease. Should our society cover or control the expense of these enhancements, or their distribution—and if so, how?

3. How should we address the new technology's "opportunity costs"—the nonmedical needs we can't fill because we keep spending so much money on health care? More of that spending in the future will be private outlays by the wealthy, leading to the further question: *Can* we address them?

4. What will be the other hidden costs of bio-, nano-, and compu-technology? How shall we foresee their social benefits and risks clearly? Can we embrace the benefits and still avoid the risks?

In Chapter 12, we considered three roads our health-care policy might take: pure retail, a national health plan, and marginal adjustments to the status quo. There's actually a fourth, although it's more of an outlook for the journey than a path per se. In 1971, a Korean War veteran, ex-professor of creative writing, and self-proclaimed hippie-beatnik named Stephen Gaskin led the founders of The Farm in Summertown, Tennessee, the most successful commune in recent American history. In 2000 he ran—or, more accurately, walked—for president of the United States. At that time he outlined his own health plan: "Let's take care of everybody now and argue about the money later." In politics these days, such an idea can come only from the fringe of the fringe, but it's as clear a statement of decent medical priorities as we're likely to find.

America will always have twinges of conscience. As we lust for flashy new tools to make ourselves healthier, wealthier, and Pfizer, we will wonder what to do for, or with, those who need medicine for illness but can't afford it. Do we just leave them in the waiting room? Do we ask government to ride in on its gray charger and make some sort of insurance bridge for the working poor, in the hope that administering the law would cost society less than footing the bill for treating these people at public clinics plus losses from their untreated illnesses? That much might be feasible toward mid-decade, with a new administration in Washington, especially if budget surpluses reappear by then. Or do we just sit tight for 20 years, hoping that the conflict between genetic antidiscrimination laws and medical costs will kill the insurance industry and force us into a national health plan for therapeutic medicine?

At present, European-style socialized medicine or a Canadian-type single-payer insurance plan seems out of the question in this country, even though a majority of Americans, when polled, say they want a national system. The very word "socialized" is a bogeyman that makes our talking heads foam at the mouth. And the United States indeed may be too large and diverse for any one-size-fits-all solution to work, no matter how well administered.

Redefining Health

One of the great truths that gets overlooked in the rush to develop genetic medicine is the fact that health is something other than, and greater than, all the medical technology ever developed or yet to come.

This is the traditional outlook encoded in the very language we speak. The word "health" comes via German from the Indo-European root *kailo,* meaning both whole and holy. "Doctor" derives from words for "teach" in Latin and Greek. "Medicine" descends from the Indo-European *med-,* to take proper measures, pausing in Greek to give us Medusa, the witch-healer whose serpent hair slithered to Eden's tree of good and evil and the doctor's staff of life and death. Thus etymology tells us that a true health-care practitioner is "a teacher who takes appropriate measures to make whole."

If so, then medicine must be a branch of philosophy, the art of living. It might be called the *physical* art of living. If that is true, then medicine run only as a business will surely fail, no matter how potent its techniques. It will be at cross-purposes with life, which follows a different logic than money does.

If, on the other hand, medicine is nothing more than a system of technical expertise, then we really don't need the concept of health at all. The body will be declared incompetent and committed to become a ward of that modern meta-body, the corp-oration. The entire $2 trillion enterprise will be reduced to a game in which "we" (all of us) tacitly agree to bring every problem or need to medicine in order that "we" (a few of us) may profit from solving the problem or filling the need.

The second, narrower definition is the one we in the United States keep choosing, and it produces what we have today: detailed management of the individual concerns of people with the money, time, and savvy to work the system. This approach crowds out prevention, education, self-care, community medicine, and other ways of cheaply promoting health en masse, just as junk food crowds nutrients out of the diet. The factor most important to health, prevention, gets less than five cents of our medical dollar.

The difficulty is not so much that medicine is overpriced, though it is. But the cost is only a symptom. The real problem is that there's far too *much* medicine, an oversupply to which we've become addicted. We rely on it far more than any society ever has before, and we accrue far too little health in return for our staggering investment. When we examine medicine with a clinical eye, we find that it makes a surprisingly small contribution to our health. We see that our blind faith in it infantilizes us, weakening the sense of major accountability for our own health that is a mark of adulthood.

Curative power is a wonderful thing, but the fact is: *Medicine does not create health*. We are in danger of making that old mistake in a new era. As two doctors, Neil A. Holtzman and Theresa M. Marteau, recently reminded their peers:

> In our rush to fit medicine with the genetic mantle, we are
> losing sight of other possibilities for improving the public
> health. Differences in social structure, lifestyle, and environ-
> ment account for much larger proportions of disease than
> genetic differences.

Health is largely the product and by-product of self-knowledge and responsible living. It comes from prudent social investment in a clean environment, from vigorous communities that can ensure safe streets without martial law, from loving and well-informed families, from tolerant acceptance of human physical and mental diversity, as well as from an efficient medical system that works when called upon but doesn't burden us unduly.

To avoid feeling overwhelmed by the wrong problem, we must keep in view the context of medicine's dilemma. It is like the world's plight in many ways. Humans, primarily the Western, Indo-European strain, have proliferated under the social order called capitalism. In so doing, they have:

- Used up most of the treasure of fossil fuel laid down in the Carboniferous Era
- Thereby produced global warming and the consequent floods and droughts that will bedevil the earth for the next century or millennium
- Annihilated, intentionally or by reckless disregard, much of the living natural world, including the human world, whose diversity is the legacy all previous beings have left us and the foundation upon which our own life rests—not to mention that we have thus violated these beings' innate right to life

Surely the impact of these choices on human health is far greater than that of any tinkering we may now do with the U.S. medical-care system.

Those who wish to think constructively about health care must recognize, first of all, that anything we do to reform it will have only marginal effects until we somehow alter a central aspect of our entire civilization, its rapacity. For that, too, is at the core of our economics—a Greek word meaning "house rules." The object of the capitalist game, stripped to its essentials, is to *capitalize* on one another's mistakes, weaknesses, needs, fears, hungers—even to trash the earth if there's a buck in it. Apparently we are unable to regulate industry to save the ozone layer, but members of the Western middle and upper classes will soon have ultraviolet skin-patch dosimeters to warn them if they get too much sun.

This is libertarian individualism flipped into some hyperspace parody of itself. It ignores the deeper truth that the sacred individual can fully flourish only within a community, that the best ideology might be libertarian communitarianism, a "both . . . and" society in which rights and duties are in balance at the point where one's own actions impinge on others, in which the urge to give back proceeds naturally from tolerant, beneficent governance.

Our welfare programs and safety nets are laudable attempts to mitigate our social system's essential cruelty. But they're downstream fixes for an upstream problem. That's why they're so complex and work so poorly.

On the contrary, deep within us we each carry the certainty, acknowledged or not, that we are most emphatically *not* all in it together, that in fact it is every man, woman, child, beast, and tree for itself.

Moreover, we like to think that, even if our time is lonely, at least it's our own. Laboriously we have ground our standard workweek down from a robber-baronial 60 or 70 hours to 35 or 40. That's what can be legally required in a union job. The actual average, says the Families and Work Institute, is 49 hours for men and 42 for women. Not counting commute, shopping, housework, and so on.

Americans, on average, get almost two hours less sleep per night than we did even a century ago. Most of us manage only half an hour a week for sexual activity, yet we tsk-tsk about the desire for drugs to support and enhance our sexuality. Compare all that with a workweek of 18 to 24 hours in so-called primitive societies.

We in the modern world are told that we all have a lot of disposable time. In fact, most of our time is at the disposal of others. The resultant fatigue, isolation, anxiety, depression—many of the givens in our daily lives—have severe medical consequences that are rarely considered.

Are these broader social, political, and economic issues relevant in a book about the promise and peril of the new medicine? Yes, profoundly so. In the long run, we will find that we cannot have a healthy medicine in a sick society.

The *Yuck* Factor

We have mentioned socialized medicine, a health-care system whose role as servant of all citizens is defined by law. But constructive authority also might flow the other way, from medicine to society. An effective social medicine of the future might concern itself with the social conditions truly required for well-being, instead of just trimming the cogs to fit the wheels.

Such a meta-medicine would take an active role in opposing cultural root causes of disease, like extreme disparities of wealth, the overfeeding industry, and the beating and sexual abuse of children. It would demand an end to the prosecution of those who commit victimless crimes and offer real help to addicts. In schools, it might promote recess over Ritalin. Genetic study of chimpanzee, gorilla, and human sperm has shown that throughout nearly all of our 2 million–year history humans have lived in great sexual freedom, what some would call promiscuity. Confirmation of this primordial birthright could lead to a prescription for more loving and less damning. If health care stays aloof from such social issues, it may gain skill at treating the results, but it will be helpless to prevent them.

In addition, our standard philosophy of health rarely considers social problems caused *by* medicine. We have discussed economic class divisions likely to be worsened by the retail market in genetic enhancements. We've mentioned the danger that parental selection of their offspring's gender may skew the ratio of women to men. But genetic medicine may produce an even more radical shift in sexual politics.

Priests got rid of priestesses by making God a sexless man. Doctors ousted midwives by medicalizing birth. In like manner, now every molecular detail of human reproduction seems destined to become mediated through a class of gene-priests who are overwhelmingly male. Though not consciously intended as such, this development could be the ultimate usurpation of women's status and biological function. Its prevention would require restrictions on medicine, or forbearance within it, neither of which seems likely in the near future.

But attitudes can change. We may come to require more social accountability from the health-care industry. Genomic medicine might even be the occasion for such a shift. But so far, many of the efforts toward that end seem strangely off point.

There is a powerful instinctive *yuck* factor in many people's reactions to genetic manipulation. Vegetarians, of whom there are at least a billion on earth, will object to implanting animal genes in plants. It's too bad that some Christian fundamentalists are trying to harness the yuck factor in their fight to unteach evolution and withdraw abortion rights from women. Hitching fears about biotechnology to those creaky wagons could end up making "the public" seem so irrational that science will become *less* willing to be accountable to it.

Shortsighted pressure from organized religion can make things worse, even from its own point of view. A case in point is the pressure that a coalition of Christian churches brought to bear on the American Cancer Society in 2000. The churches convinced the ACS to withdraw from Patients for CURE, a group supporting stem-cell research, by threatening to end church-group donations, which form a big chunk of the ACS's annual half billion dollars in income from gifts. In the end, such blackmail can only drive research more firmly into the corporate embrace and further from any public control.

In terms of medicine's future, there are at least two more things wrong with the religious response to genetic medicine so far.

First, much of organized religion asks us to care more about surplus zygotes than people who are walking around, hoping for a cancer cure. And naturally enough: If Saint Peter awaits with eternal life at the pearly gates, then the world before birth and after death is the only one that matters. But for those unwilling to put all their eggs in the Easter basket, it's what's *between* birth and death that counts. Mutual understanding will require some "both. . . and" thinking from each side, but it will be hard to form alliances across that gap.

Second—and polarizing the debate even more—churchly opposition to all study of human embryos reenacts the tired old play of orthodoxy trying to prevent the expansion of knowledge. Blotchy woodcuts of Urban VIII, Bishop Wilberforce, and William Jennings Bryan flit across our minds, and suddenly all doubt about the unlimited advance of science seems reactionary.

But people's queasiness is actually nonsectarian. Furthermore, religious feelings about the sanctity of life merit respect in their own right. Shorn of narrow political agendas, such feelings might unite not only America's increasingly diverse Christians but also the growing numbers of non-Christians, agnostics, and atheists as well. Such unity could be a crucial brake on unregulated trade in living materials.

Even though the benefits of genetic medicine sound great, many of us feel in our guts that we're crossing dangerous lines too fast, with too little understanding of the consequences—too little self-knowledge as well as scientific knowledge. Even if we are ready technologically, emotionally we're children playing with really big matches. We rightly fear mishandling life like incompetent programmers who ruin good software by introducing snazzy subroutines without understanding the whole program. A few genetic *Exxon Valdez*'s could create the climate for a tighter rein on medical research, or all biotechnology.

Toward a More Humane Medicine

Barring such disasters, there may still be ways to control the biomedical complex and redirect biotech medicine along more humane lines.

One of them might be to require such stringent testing and high licensing fees that certain areas of development become unprofitable. Certainly the industry needs regulating, and enforcement, as the death of young Jesse Gelsinger from an untested genetic medicine showed. But relying primarily on government rules is problematic. For one thing, it's reactive. Rules generally get made only in response to abuses that are already well established, and therefore hard to eradicate. Furthermore, it's hard to see future problems in detail; without proactive safeguards, horses are always escaping from barns before the doors can be shut.

For another thing, the biotech industry is already huge and will grow exponentially in the next few decades. No single agency can police it all, especially with the lobbying power it will possess to shrink regulatory budgets and weaken mandates. Trying to make biotechnology subject to specific kinds of damage assessments in civil law could lead to legislation exempting it from *all* liability—a genetic version of the Price-Anderson Act of 1957, which protects the nuclear business from liability. In the event of a really major gray-goo faux pas, who'd be around to collect anyway?

The biotech industry already has shown itself to be supremely focused on channeling money toward its own expansion at the expense of broader concerns. At its BIO2000 conference in Boston in March 2000, Biotechnology Industry Association reps crowed about raising $8 billion of research funds in the previous three months. Then they gave the keynote speaker, Christopher Reeve, an amazingly chintzy $5,000 check for his paralysis foundation. If Congress can't limit the corporate right to hawk sugar-plated starch bullets to kids, how in the world is it going to protect us against sweet-tooth genes or chromosomal lemons from this new powerhouse?

Furthermore, overreliance on rules makes government the adversary of industry. The fact that industry's agenda is often inimical to the public good is all the more reason for government to try to avoid having such a powerful enemy. Decades of largely ineffectual attempts to legislate environmental sanity teach a sobering lesson on this point.

One approach might be to cultivate an altruistic strain in business. (We'll pause here until the laughter dies down.)

Actually, medicine's history as a service profession should make it more susceptible than most industries to such an approach. Some of its corporate leaders already are trying to rise to the challenge.

Drug companies often follow this maxim: Try it on the poor, sell it to the rich. The vaccine for hepatitis B was tested on the people of Senegal, but they can't afford the finished product. By the same token, there's no paying market to call forth an effective drug or vaccine for malaria or sleeping sickness.

Now, however, the AIDS vaccine developed by France's Pasteur Merieux company is being tested in Uganda with the understanding that, if successful, it will be distributed there at subsidized prices. Through the Gates Foundation, Bill Gates has begun a program to buy the hepatitis B vaccine, as well as the one for *Hemophilus influenzae* type b, and distribute them in the Third World at nominal rates. By joining with other philanthropies, he hopes to create a guaranteed market to encourage pharmaceutical research on diseases prevalent in the poorest nations.

SmithKline directors recently showed how it's done by announcing the donation of 20 billion doses of their drug albendazole, used for treating the intestinal parasites that cause elephantiasis, to Third World nations in an attempt to eradicate the disease within two decades. The small programs under which several drug companies now donate medicines to community health centers for the uninsured poor could be expanded considerably, both in this country and abroad.

AstraZeneca announced in May 2000 that it will give away seed for its golden rice free to developing nations, helped along by patent holders' relinquishment of royalties for such donations. This is a rice engineered with genes from daffodils and a bacterium to produce beta-carotene (provitamin A). It is expected to be ready for market in 2003. Proponents hope that it may prevent 2 million infant deaths and a half million cases of blindness from vitamin A deficiency each year.

It should be noted, however, that a diet adequate in fat and protein is required for full utilization of vitamin A; thus, it remains to be seen whether this gesture will really help those who need it most. Will we say it's the thought that counts? Such initiatives may be the start of a trend toward apple polishing by the biotechnology industry—striving to gain a reputation for having a social conscience without actually undertaking the genuine measures that would demonstrate the substance of one. Everyone who cares about the problem of hunger knows the real reason the Third World can't feed itself: Its landless peasants have to grow coffee and McCattle to make export profits for its landowning elites, who are kept in place by Western economic interests. Giving away golden-rice seeds will not solve the central faults of our global economic system, but the gift may help, and it certainly won't make the problems worse.

Most corporations are concerned about their image, and advocacy advertising might have great impact by publicizing those that do and those that do not give something back to the world they profit from. Thus, isolated acts of corporate generosity might combine and grow into a movement fostering true concern for the welfare of the earth on the part of every company—a sort of Hippocratic oath for business. In any case, the degree to which the biotechnology powers try to colonize life and continue corporate patterns of exploitation will determine much about the future. Under Mikhail Gorbachev, the Soviets belatedly tried "communism with a human face." At a much earlier stage of a new historical process, "capitalism with a human face" might do a lot to smooth out the upheavals of the genetic revolution.

Social medicine could be a powerful ally for progress. The problems that physicians face in their newly mercantile profession might lead to a new activism on their part, and the trend toward medicalization might make our leaders ready to listen.

In society's consulting room, we might be able to consider the health of the polity in such matters as victimless crime or the two extremes of sexual repression and trivialization. We could consider treating absent-father syndrome with flexible work options, day-care subsidies, and equalized custody and visitation laws. We might follow the etiology of adult sexual predation back to our chronic plague of child beating and molestation, thus lowering the costs of depression, obesity, and addiction as well. The day might come when authoritarian religious mania might be treatable, like any other mental illness, and rigid religious indoctrination of the young might be considered another form of child abuse.

Under the tutelage of an enlightened medical science our social minds might expand to include such ideas as *soul*—not the death survivor we all dream of but rather what black people often mean by the term: juice, joie de vivre, the generous exuberant spirit of a person fully alive in *this* world. (Isn't that the very quality our geneticists claim to be seeking the secret to?)

Are we wandering off the subject here? We think not. The Declaration of Independence guarantees us the right to pursue happiness, but capitalism demands that we endlessly gain a purchase, yet never quite grasp it. In the end, to speak realistically about reducing medical costs, one must think idealistically about a society in which we—the real we, nearly all of us or as close to all as we can get—are happy.

In that visionary state, we would not be in constant overstressed pursuit, not be driven from inside or out. We'd be unburdened from the world's 450 billionaires, who own more than all put together of the world's poorest half, numbering 3 billion people. Wages everywhere suddenly would exceed the cost of living by a comfortable margin. Schools would have resources to match their students, and all students would have a future to prepare for. No longer would conditions in the inner cities make armed robbery look like a promising career choice. Financial barriers to food distribution and doctrinal barriers to population control would fall, ending the mass starvation that is our system's greatest crime. Most of us could look forward as children to a life of satisfying work and a good chance of romantic fulfillment, connected to family, friends, community, and the earth.

In a word, happy. And thereby healthy. Think about the need for medicine in such a place. Visualize the whole monstrous apparatus of today's health-care industry dwindling into an efficient medical profession superbly accomplished at therapeutics and overseeing with rigorous care the elective fruits of our genetic labors. Think of a health-care system with its prowess enhanced and its mission restored but costing us much less, one half or even one third of what it does today.

If we the people hope to get even part of the way from here to there, we must try to avoid lapsing into a reflexive, defeatist quietism. Instead, we need to support the efforts of any friends we may find among corporate officers, legislators, and entrepreneurial scientists. But we certainly can't leave it all up to them. If even the best of them seem helpless against a horrendous future, what can the rest of us do?

Allies in the Struggle

We might start by reminding ourselves that we have two allies in which we can place great faith. One is our own innate skepticism, our sense of rightness, especially when combined with the energy of youth. It is emerging again in protests against global-ism's inequities and iniquities. If somehow we can route that energy around the *Six O'clock News* and amplify it through uncontrolled media, it might grow into something earth-shaking—not earth-shaking from the self-defeating violence of terrorist theocracies but instead perhaps from a World Strike or a new round of Velvet Revolutions.

Our second ally is nature, the indifferent yet supportive matrix of all life. It is weak under assault but has great endurance and is noted for comebacks against long odds. It is the green shoot forcing its way through concrete. Remembering the resilience of natural life can reassure us that it's not all up to us. With help, nature has saved Americans from the embarrassment of killing off the bald eagle and thereby having an extinct national emblem.

The law is sometimes agonizingly slow to make obviously needed changes, but its natural conservatism also might work in our favor. A movement among lawyers to promote social responsibility could certainly be a powerful force for constructive change.

Some expect the Web to help us save ourselves, or at least save money on medicine. Several companies now offer full-scale peer-reviewed medical briefings for laypersons on all but the most esoteric ailments. For less serious conditions, these can sometimes replace an office visit. Often they serve as a preconsultation, helping the patient be prepared with questions and a basic knowledge of the problem, and so make best use of the physician's time.

The Web is ideal for other kinds of information, too. Cancer patients and their doctors often used to have a hard time finding out about experimental treatments, but a recently opened National Cancer Institute site keeps a database of clinical trials, updated daily. At least one company, started by one of the authors

(Carlson), helps people retrieve, collate, understand, correct, and archive their medical records, much like services that let people take control of their credit records.

By helping people gather and assimilate information for themselves, the Web may be a great leveler. It still needs better filters to sift the vast and fast-growing amount of data, varying widely in quality, for what's relevant—especially when the seeker doesn't yet know exactly what he's seeking. Most folks don't have time to grind through five thousand hits in search of the few they need.

And the Web may hold down medical spending a little, in two ways: by letting us comparison-shop before making the first appointment, and by empowering low-tech self-help alternatives to avoid more expensive options. On the other hand, holistic medicine and its associated health-food and supplements market may remain mostly a prerogative of the well-off and information-rich, just as President Reagan, through his administration's policies of deregulation, encouraged food makers to treat the meat of the Great Unwashed however they pleased, while he himself dined on strictly organic beef hand-raised on his ranch.

Like most technology, the Web may end up having an equivocal effect. One fear is that fee-based sites might re-create the drawbacks of proprietary databases, becoming too expensive for most individuals. The opposite danger is a trend toward sites so choked by advertising as to make them too much trouble to use.

The Web has enormous potential for control as well as for freedom. Consider the FBI's Carnivore, a customized packet sniffer, a program that searches through electronic traffic in search of any word or phrase sought by the operator. No consent of the Internet service provider is required for it to be installed on an e-mail server. Once activated, it can sort out all messages containing keywords—for example, slang terms for a prohibited drug or the name of someone suspected of a crime—complete with the message senders' addresses and phone numbers. The FBI promises to use it only pursuant to a court-ordered e-mail wiretap against a specific ISP customer suspected of using the Internet for illegal activities, and the Bureau recently hired a former Justice Department official to check and make sure that that was all the software was doing.

Believable? Your call. We're dubious, especially in today's post–September 11 world, in which the antiterrorist cause has been enlisted in support of all manner of assaults on civil liberties.

The inability of law enforcers to abide by the law is justly proverbial, and often expensive. Even Plato couldn't figure out who would police the police themselves.

One thing is certain: There'll be a steady market for anonymizing and encryption software. Programmers and users will try to stay one jump ahead in a new race between cop cats and people mice. With luck, the Internet will become a long-term ally in the fight for more humane uses of technology.

The Short-Term Forecast: Rough Sailing

Is there any way out?

The short answer: No.

There is no tendency, ploy, or strategy on the horizon that seems likely to save us from paying any of the prices of politicized, capitalized biotech medicine, whether they be fiscal, social, or ecological costs. Naive as it sounds, our best long-term hope may be public awareness of what overreliance on technology does to us, so that a desire for economy and restraint may help counterbalance the worship of the Wholly Buyable. We happen to believe that an informed public is the ultimate public good.

The new-medicine revolution is proceeding with a certainty that is purely technical, and illusory at that. To date, there is no credible effort to ensure cumulative ecological safety from all the genetically engineered product organisms entering the biosphere. The $3 million that scientists thought would suffice to get answers to the question of whether Bt corn pollen kills monarch butterflies in the wild has turned out to be inadequate. Yet that amount is three times the Agriculture Department's annual budget for *all* ecosafety testing.

Trying to answer thousands of such questions on a case-by-case basis, even if it were possible, still would ignore the complexity of real-world multispecies interdependence. The piecemeal, downstream approach also ignores the fact that environmental innovations often don't show their full consequences for 50 or 100 years, or more. Even so, the chief of the Biotechnology Industry Organization's food and agriculture division, Michael Phillips, has warned us all not to expect corporations to address the issue in any meaningful way.

Resistance on the part of the industry to informative labeling proves that the industry itself has no faith whatsoever in the long-term safety of its products. If it did, it would label them proudly, rather than hiding behind the FDA's skirts. Companies would vie with each other in giving complete accounts of the transformations involved in creating their products. Instead, most of us don't know exactly what we're eating. In a poll conducted by the American Museum of Natural History in conjunction with its "Genomic Revolution" exhibit in the summer of 2001, 70 percent of respondents said they had never eaten genetically modified food. The Union of Concerned Scientists estimates, to the contrary, that half of all processed food in the country contains at least one GM ingredient.

If guided only by lemming capital, one day this industry will rush us all over a cliff of carelessness or cruelty into a sea of trouble. It matters not whether the specifics be a sudden plague or simply a long slide into a world even more stratified than the one we live in, full of wonders yet so much less free, so much harsher and shabbier for most than it might have been.

What gets controlled, people or technology? Can quaint old "enlightened public opinion" really jump the runaway biotech train and keep it on the rails? Let's find out! Protests at home helped keep Johnson and Nixon from pursuing the Vietnam War to extermination. Electronic media helped mobilize Velvet Revolutions in South Africa, the Philippines, and the entire Soviet empire. To assume that we are powerless is to be so.

How to Fix the System

All of us—including policy pundits who have any influence in the real world, leaders of courage within science and business, a few lawmakers free of donor puppet strings, people of goodwill who might form a mass movement—all of us will have to unite long enough to fix our health-care system in the only way it can stay fixed.

That means we fix up the neighborhood. We liberate medicine decisively from its uses as investment vehicle or arsenal. Toward that end we list here a few policy changes that will be needed as steps along the way, fully aware that enacting even one or two of them will require Herculean political labors:

- *Rescind the patentability of genes and living organisms, both natural and artificial.* That's the one giveaway that is set to cause our worst problems in the twenty-first century. The giveback is the one act of good faith on the part of biotechnology that can call forth equal good faith from the people, so as to write a new social contract in the new era.
- *In return, protect biological inventors with more traditional use-patents or patents on procedures.* Model these exclusivity provisions on those of the Orphan Drug Act.
- *Require that every patent for a process using naturally occurring genetic material must include cash royalties or equivalent compensation for the people or land from which the plasm originates.*
- *Likewise require that a patent for a product likely to diminish people's livelihoods must include generous assistance for their transition to another source of income.*
- *Once and for all, make access to therapeutic medicine a right, not a privilege.* Guarantee that therapeutic medicine should be available at cost, not as a profit-generating machine with a multitiered bureaucratic equivalent of the risk investors raking in their 30 percent off the top. Then hammer out the best compromises we can on equal access to nontherapeutic upgrade medicine, as much by consensus as possible.
- *Politically engineer activist strains of medicine, science, and business to make common cause with people in their effort to repeal victimless crimes.* This will lower medical costs and restore trust in the police by focusing their undivided attention on fraud, theft, rape, murder, and other true crimes.

- *Enlist all possible allies to eliminate the secret branches of the United States government, or at least to prevent their access to genetic technology.* This is perhaps the most important change required of Americans before the rest of the world can live with us in peace.
- *Develop a socially responsible specialty within medicine to oversee an extremely cautious insertion of genetic changes into the ecosystem.* In the final analysis, biotransformations of our food and manufactured goods are medical procedures with potentially catastrophic medical consequences. Before it's too late, we must counterbalance the profit stampede by insisting on strict observance of Hippocrates' cardinal rule: First, do no harm. In law, the legal fiction of a corporation should have no more rights than a person, especially when it comes to subjecting us all to an experiment.
- *Establish an international authority to inspect and enforce a moratorium on specified research.* This program could be based on the two-year abstention from recombinant DNA work agreed to by geneticists at the 1975 Asilomar Conference.

To expand on the last point above: Some procedures, like nuclear power generation, are so inherently dangerous that they must be done *infallibly*. But the assumption that humans can be infallible is absurd. Where the stakes are too high for mistakes, development must not proceed at all, ever.

The enforcement body must be composed primarily of ordinary citizens and environmentalists. Representatives of government, science, and business *must not* have a majority, or it will be useless.

As for Monsanto, some suggest that the company should be seized and that half its assets should be divided among its victims; the other half should go to reimburse its shareholders as well as may be; and that its directors should be given 10 to 20 years—in Leavenworth, not Allenwood.

Seen from a moral perspective, the company and its executives may well deserve such treatment. Nevertheless, Monsanto's actions, though offensive, are not clearly defined as crimes in most nations. Such legal definition is an essential first step toward accountability for environmental consequences of biotechnological tinkering. If the citizenry ever has enough power to punish Fortune 500 executives, we suggest that pardons for past actions might be useful bargaining chips to negotiate economic concessions.

In any event, the levels of fines and jail terms for corporate malfeasance levied by the international and national legal systems need to be drastically revised upward. The pot of gold at the end of the genetic rainbow has called forth enormous inventiveness in making new drugs and organisms. There will be no equivalent creativity applied to safety unless we rig incentives for it. The possibility of hard time for business felons could do a lot to foster social accountability and could also spur a much-needed dismantling of the inhuman prison racket that ensnares so many perpetrators of victimless crimes.

If we can help physicians return honor and sanity to their profession, they may lead us into an earthly Oz, there to live as did the gods of old. The ancient Greek poet Hesiod divined the life span of dryads, the guardian spirits of the woods, to be about 300,000 years, which is a pretty good approximation of the death and rebirth of forests during the most recent ice ages. Most of us would be quite pleased even with our estimated telomere-programmed limit of 120 years in full.

Many ancient and medieval societies were built on a form of genetic determinism, called aristocracy. Those with the best "blood" inherited the top positions in society and also got preferential treatment from religion when it came to entering paradise and enjoying the afterlife. The pyramid builders and cathedral masons tried to ensure immortality for the pharaoh and his court, and for the cathedral's noble patrons. Today it seems that one of the main goals of our medical system will be longevity, an on-ramp to immortality, for the richest and most powerful members of our society—the top of the pyramid.

In most cultures known to history, the anonymous majority have lived their lives vicariously through what the historian Milton Klonsky called the "fabulous ego" of the king, the aristocrats, the rich and famous, the movie stars. We like to think our world is better. We like to think that, if our society is often unfair, it has at least given many of its members a chance to succeed on their own terms. But now our health-care system, one of our proudest creations, which we meant to be available to all, by its unparalleled success may be leading us backward into a brave old future too much like the past for comfort.

It doesn't have to be that way. Besides fabulous egos, history is also littered with defeated giants who once seemed invincible. If together we muster the will to tame genetic medicine on a cooperative worldwide basis, we can give our descendants a bright future—a more egalitarian society glowing with health and using its new understanding of life wisely.

Notes

Chapter 2: Too Much of a Good Thing

36 **health-care fraud estimate of $100 billion:** Gauged at $80 billion 10 years ago by Gordon Witkin with Dorian Friedman and Monika Guttman, "Health Care Fraud," *U.S. News & World Report,* 24 February 1992.

36 **administrative expenses:** During the reform push, *Consumer Reports* estimated the price of management at $163 billion, one fifth of all medical costs, and found half of it utterly unnecessary. See "Wasted Health Care Dollars," *Consumer Reports,* July 1992.

46 **doubled consumption of goods and services:** Dawn Stover, "6 Billion and Counting," *Popular Science,* October 1999, p. 39, reported these statistics as the human population passed 6 billion.

47 **private study of longevity trends:** Lee Bowman, "New Study Suggests People Will Live Even Longer in the Future," Scripps Howard News Service, 24 June 2000, summarized a study by Shripad Tuljapurkar, Nan Li, and Carol Boe, "A Universal Pattern of Mortality Decline in the G7 Countries," *Nature* 405 (20 June 2000): 789–792.

48 **future demand for nursing homes:** "Projected Health Conditions Among the Elderly," http://www.aoa.dhhs.gov/aoa/stats/aging21.

54 **"medical losses" by for-profits and nonprofits:** Nancy Ann Jeffrey, "For-Profit HMOs Deliver Worse Care Than Not-for-Profit

Plans, Study Finds," *Wall Street Journal,* 14 July 1999, is a report of a study by David Himmelstein, Steffie Woolhandler, Ida Hellander, and Sidney Wolfe, "Quality of Care in Investor-Owned vs. Not-for-Profit HMOs," *Journal of the American Medical Association* 282 (14 July 1999): 159.

55 deaths from medication errors: David Phillips, professor of sociology at University of California–San Diego in La Jolla, cited in Harper's Index, March 1998.

60 insurer donations to Ways and Means Committee: *Playboy,* Significa, April 1994.

60 Packwood's "fingerprints": Senator Bob Packwood, in an address to party colleagues over lunch in Washington, D.C., on September 13, 1994. Three days later, in reply to a reporter who asked whether he really made this remark, Packwood said, "I don't know. I don't remember what I say from one day to the next."

61 "common in the industry": Kurt Eichenwald, "He Blew the Whistle, and Health Giants Quaked," *New York Times,* 18 October 1998, A1.

Chapter 3: Gold in Them Thar Ills

66 market for artificial skin: David J. Mooney and Antonios Mikos, "Growing New Organs," *Scientific American,* April 1999.

70 price rises in corporate medical plans: N. R. Kleinfield, "Life, Death, and Managed Care," *New York Times,* 14 November 1999, A1, summarizes several years of findings published in the "Hewitt Health Value Initiative," a database and annual survey of health-care plans at 300 large corporations, compiled by Hewitt Associates, Lincolnshire, Ill. Hewitt forecasts 13 to 16 percent increases in average medical-plan costs for 2002.

70 inflation in prescription plans: Watson Wyatt Worldwide,

Health Care Costs 2002 (Bethesda, Md.: Watson Wyatt World-wide, 2001), an annual survey of 200 corporations, projects drug-plan cost hikes of nearly 20 percent in 2002.

75 **Granddad's cholesterol-control drug:** Maybe he should just stop worrying about cholesterol, which George Mann, former codirector of the Framingham Study, calls "the greatest health scam of the century." But that's another story.

77 **children losing Medicaid benefits in cutbacks:** Robert Pear, "A Million Parents Lost Medicaid, Study Says," *New York Times*, 19 June 2000, reports a study by Families USA.

77 **redumping of Medicare patients:** Nancy Ann Jeffrey, "Who's Crowding E.R.s Now? Managed-Care Patients," *Wall Street Journal*, 29 July 1999, A1.

Chapter 4: Market *über Alles*

80 **advertising's role in drug-cost increases:** Steven D. Findlay, *Prescription Drugs and Mass Media Advertising 2000* (Washington, D.C.: National Institute for Health Care Management, 2001). Since 1993, four classes of drugs—antihistamines, cholesterol reducers, ulcer remedies, and antidepressants—accounted for the largest share of the increase in drug costs. The same four groups also have accounted for the largest share of direct-to-consumer advertising since its legalization in 1997. In 2000 there was a 19 percent rise in retail spending on pharmaceuticals. Most of it resulted from an increase in the number of prescriptions rather than in drug-price increases. The 50 most heavily advertised drugs were prescribed 25 percent more often that year than the previous year; the other 9,850 drugs were prescribed only 4 percent more often.

85 **Mark Taylor's therapeutic mattress:** Andrew Goldstein, "Never Again," *Time*, 20 December 1999, 53.

85 physicians fighting to regain control: See, for example, Katherine Eban Finkelstein, "Rebels in White Coats," *Nation,* 21 February 2000.

87 HMOs' public-confidence rating: Just 17 percent, according to a Gallup–USA Today–CNN poll taken June 25–27, 1999.

88 denial-of-coverage appeals: Michael M. Weinstein, "Managed Care's Other Problem: It's Not What You Think," *New York Times,* 7 March 1999.

Chapter 5: A Patent Misunderstanding

108 too risky to proceed: As a result of the Gelsinger tragedy, the watchdog powers of the RAC, which had been weakened and shifted to the FDA, have been restored.

112 quote by Patrick Brown: Kristen Philipkoski, "Science + Business: A Bad Mix?" *Wired* News, 18 February 2000.

Chapter 6: False Profits

121 charges unrelated to patient care: "Scams: What Medicare Covers," *Harper's,* November 1996, 32.

121 Ted Fishman's fraud research: Ted Fishman, "Up in Smoke: The Suckers Bring the Money; Wall Street Supplies the Matches," *Harper's,* December 1998.

122 the take from Vitamins Inc.: David Barboza, "Tearing Down the Facade of 'Vitamins Inc.,' " *New York Times,* 10 October 1999.

123 quashing the Remune report: Philip J. Hilts, "Company Tried to Bar Report That H.I.V. Vaccine Failed," *New York Times,* 1 November 2000.

Chapter 8: Personal Alchemy

145 best plastic surgeons salvaging work of the worst: Estimate of Dr. Gerald Pitman, quoted in Claudia Kalb, "Our Quest to Be Perfect," *Newsweek,* 9 August 1999, 58.

149 synaptic patterns of fear: For a short summary of recent discoveries, written for the lay reader, see Stephen S. Hall, "Fear Itself," *New York Times Magazine,* 28 February 1999.

152 gratitude to the pharmaceutical companies: Kelly Luker, "At Peace with Prozac," *Salon.com,* 17 May 2000.

Chapter 9: Living Commodities

158 fertility clinic egg thieves: Suzanne Goldenberg, "Doctors Accused of Stealing Human Eggs," *Guardian,* 19 May 2000.

158 bidding on supermodel eggs: "Auction Begins for Models' Eggs," reported on MSNBC News online, 25 October 1999.

163 wrongful-birth suit: "Boy Compensated for Being Born," Reuters, 17 November 2000.

166 A. R. Luria's memory performer: A. R. Luria, *The Mind of a Mnemonist: A Little Book About a Vast Memory,* trans. L. Solotaroff (Cambridge, Mass.: Harvard University Press, 1968).

171 seeing through a cat's eyes: David Whitehouse, "Computer Uses Cat's Brain to See," BBC News, 8 October 1999, reporting a study by Garrett Stanley, Fei Li, and Yang Dan, "Reconstruction of Natural Scenes from Ensemble Responses in the Lateral Geniculate Nucleus," *Journal of Neuroscience* 19 (September 15, 1999): 8036.

Chapter 10: Silent Bombs

185 **wheat smut and infected turkey feathers:** For an excellent overview of crop bombs, see Paul Rogers, Simon Whitby, and Malcolm Dando, "Biological Warfare Against Crops," *Scientific American*, June 1999.

186 **Iacocca's Pinto widows:** Mark Dowie, "Pinto Madness," *Mother Jones*, September–October 1977.

194 **gray-goo problem:** George B. Dyson, *Darwin Among the Machines: The Evolution of Global Intelligence* (New York: Helix Books/Perseus, 1998); Bill Joy, "Why the Future Doesn't Need Us," *Wired*, April 2000; K. Eric Drexler, *Engines of Creation: The Coming Era of Nanotechnology* (New York: Anchor/Doubleday, 1987).

196 **round heels:** For the FDA's own declaration that its mission is to "foster" biotechnology rather than regulate it, see "Genetically Engineered Foods," *FDA Consumer*, January–February 1993, 14.

Chapter 11: Everything Is Under Control

209 **a very big question:** For a cautionary corrective against millennial genomic hype, see R. L. Zimmern, "The Human Genome Project: A False Dawn?" *British Medical Journal* 319 (November 13, 1999): 1282; and Neil A. Holtzman and Theresa M. Marteau, "Will Genetics Revolutionize Medicine?" *New England Journal of Medicine* 343, no. 2 (July 13, 2000): 141.

209 **undiscovered bacteria and viruses:** This idea's foremost exponent is the Amherst biologist Paul Ewald; see Judith Hooper, "A New Germ Theory," *The Atlantic Monthly*, February 1999.

211 **delving into the Dope War:** Dozens of writers have ably deconstructed the War on Drugs. For a superbly documented study of the Drug War as Son of Vietnam, a blank check for military sup-

pression of Third World revolts, see Jonathan Marshall, *Drug Wars* (Forestville, Calif.: Cohan & Cohen, 1991). For an overview of the Drug War as a pretext to gradually set up a police state behind a bland media façade in *this* country, please see Richard Lawrence Miller, *Drug Warriors and Their Prey* (Westport, Conn.: Praeger/Greenwood), 1996; and Rodney Stich, *Drugging America: A Trojan Horse* (Alamo, Calif.: Diablo Western Press, 1999).

212 **by far the safest drug known:** Marijuana, nature's antidepressant, has the lowest potential for fatal overdose of any drug studied. Its main psychoactive ingredient, delta–9 tetrahydrocannabinol (THC), has been calculated to have a therapeutic index (TI) between 400,000 and 28,000,000. The TI is a drug's margin of safety; the higher the TI, the safer the drug. For sources of these numbers in the scientific literature, see Pat Whelan, "How Many Dosages of THC Must a Human Take to Reach the LD–50% Amount?" on Cannabis.com, posted 8 October 1999.

The TI is calculated by dividing the minimum effective dose into the LD–50, the dose at which half the lab rats die. Since a high requires 0.5 to 20 milligrams, and THC in dried herb rarely exceeds 20 percent, you'd need to ingest somewhere between two pounds and two tons of the strongest marijuana at one sitting to achieve a fatal overdose. Of course, you'd die long before then of lung shock, stomach rupture, or blood dilution, but you get the point. By comparison, alcohol's TI is about 10, and as low as 4 in some susceptible individuals. That's why the macho game of chugging a fifth so often ends in death. The TI of most medical drugs is between 5 and 100.

213 **intangible costs of the Dope War:** For an attempt to calculate them, see David Cole's *No Equal Justice* (New York: New Press, 1999). A little gem by Thomas Szasz, *Ceremonial Chemistry: The Ritual Persecution of Drugs, Addicts, and Pushers* (Garden City, N.Y.: Doubleday, 1974), remains one of the best polemics on the hypocrisy of it all.

218 **the drug-war as scapegoating:** Peter McWilliams was a prolific author who died in 1999 of AIDS-related anorexia while in jail for growing marijuana to give away to patients like him. He left us an exhaustive (700-page) yet grimly hilarious survey of the whole panoply of victimless offenses in *Ain't Nobody's Business If You Do: The Absurdity of Consensual Crimes in Our Free Society* (Los Angeles: Prelude Press, 1994).

222 **recent history:** The best survey of our secret wars abroad is probably *The CIA: A Forgotten History*, by William H. Blum (London: Zed Books, 1986), available on CD-ROM as *The CIA Papers* (Cambridge, Mass.: Chestnut/CDRP, 1993).

If you want to do some homework on the full range of federal secrets, the annotated bibliography and name index compiled by Public Information Research at http://www.pir.org is a great place to start.

Chapter 12: Medicine in the Balance

228 **largest economic entity on earth:** The global assets of the Roman Catholic church may rival those of our medical system, but papal finances are too secret for us to know for sure.

228 **all other industrialized nations:** Including Australia, Austria, Belgium, Canada, the Czech Republic, Denmark, Finland, France, Germany, Greece, Hungary, Iceland, Ireland, Italy, Japan, Korea, Luxembourg, the Netherlands, New Zealand, Norway, Portugal, Spain, Sweden, Switzerland, and the United Kingdom, according to Organization for Economic Cooperation and Development, *Health at a Glance* (Paris: Organization for Economic Cooperation and Development, 2001), a biennial compilation of health-care information from many countries.

228 **beginning of herbal medicine sixty thousand years ago:** In 1974 a body believed to be that of a Neanderthal medicine man was dis-

covered in Shanidar Cave, in the Zagros Mountains of northern Iraq. Wreaths around his body were made of cornflowers, St. Barnaby's thistle, groundsel (ragwort), grape hyacinth, horsetail, hollyhock ("poor man's aspirin"), and yarrow (the name, from Old English *gearwe,* means "healer"). All of these herbs are still used as folk medicine in modern Iraq. For an excellent account of the burial, addressed to lay readers, with a photograph, see Joseph Campbell, *The Way of the Animal Powers* (San Francisco: Alfred van der Marck Editions/Harper & Row, 1983), 53. For the archaeological report, see Ralph S. Solecki, "Shanidar IV, a Neanderthal Flower Burial in Northern Iraq," *Science* 190 (28 November 1975): 880-881.

229 **removing nature's remedies from popular choice:** The same ploy is about to be tried on a global basis under the auspices of the Codex Alimentarius, a commission of the World Trade Organization that is ostensibly concerned with food safety. Under WTO treaties that supersede national law, the commission seeks to enforce the Vitamin Directive adopted by some members of the European Union. This regulation classifies as a prescription drug any dietary supplement that contains nutrients in excess of minimal levels set in the FDA's list of Recommended Daily Allowances. Since whole foods often exceed these limits, theoretically such a law could, for example, require one to get a doctor's permission to buy a carrot.

239 **one simple clause:** Proposed by Andrew Tobias in *The Invisible Bankers: Everything the Insurance Industry Never Wanted You to Know* (New York: Simon & Schuster, 1982).

239 **the end of insurance:** "Testing Times," *Economist,* 19 October 2000, is an anonymously written essay that presents a more detailed study of this possibility.

249 **Huntington's chorea:** For a more complete explication of this disease for the layperson, see Chapter 4 of Matt Ridley, *Genome: The Autobiography of a Species in 23 Chapters* (New York: HarperCollins, 1999).

250 **animals that still presume to eat one of us:** The feminist philosopher Val Plumwood posits grave damage to our species' mental health as a result of our refusal to be food. After barely surviving a crocodile attack in Australia's Kakadu National Park, she dissuaded park rangers from a punitive slaughter, then wrote about the experience in *The Ultimate Journey* (San Francisco: Traveler's Tales, 1999), excerpted in *Utne Reader*, July–August 2000.

251 **Sabin-vaccine contamination theory of AIDS:** Edward Hooper, *The River* (Boston: Little, Brown, 1999). Evidence presented to the Royal Society in November 2000, including genetic studies of HIV evolution, showed this theory to be unlikely though not conclusively disproved. See also Joan Stephenson, "AIDS–Polio Vaccine Link Refuted," *Journal of the American Medical Association* 285 (9 May 2001): 2319.

251 **Salk-vaccine contamination theory of mesothelioma:** Debbie Bookchin and Jim Schumacher, "The Virus and the Vaccine," *The Atlantic Monthly*, February 2000, 68–80.

Chapter 13: The Ends of Medicine

259 **fitting medicine with a genetic mantle:** Neil A. Holtzman and Theresa M. Marteau, "Will Genetics Revolutionize Medicine?" *New England Journal of Medicine* 343, no. 2 (July 13, 2000): 141.

261 **two hours less sleep per night:** For a scholarly yet readable study of exhaustion, try Juliet B. Schor, *The Overworked American: The Unexpected Decline of Leisure* (New York: Basic Books/HarperCollins, 1992).

261 **so-called primitive societies:** We call ours a leisure society, yet the anthropologist Marshall Sahlins has posited otherwise as a result of studying the work habits of various surviving "primitive"

peoples. See his essay "The Original Affluent Society," in Sahlins, *Stone Age Economics* (Chicago: Aldine, 1972).

Sahlins found that all pre-agrarian peoples worked part time, an average of 18 to 24 hours per week. The women spent 3 or 4 hours every day on food gathering and child tending combined. The men spent three or four full days a week hunting. Possessions were considered a hindrance to the primary requirement of human life in the wild—freedom of movement. Both sexes spent their abundant free time sleeping, dancing, playing, and making art and love.

262 **primordial promiscuity:** Chung-I Wu and his colleagues at the University of Chicago recently confirmed many cultures' myths and the findings of anthropologists by presenting strong evidence that prehistoric women generally showed great sexual generosity toward men. See Nicholas Wade, "DNA Data Suggest Sperm in Competition for Mating," *New York Times*, 21 January 2000, and ibid., "Battle of the Sexes Is Discerned in Sperm," *New York Times*, 22 February 2000.

The researchers studied several genes, including two for protamines, a sort of bubble-wrap that protects the fragile DNA in sperm. They found that human protamines have evolved fast, like those of chimpanzees, who mate freely, and in contrast to the slowly changing protamines of gorillas, who mate in a harem system, in which one alpha male hoards all local females.

All such genes studied so far indicate that human sperm cells have evolved to compete with other men's sperm in the vagina. They vie in terms of number, endurance, and "hard-headedness." Moreover, according to the English researcher Dr. Robin Baker of the School of Biological Sciences at the University of Manchester, there is evidence that sperm cells from each man display a sort of "team spirit," aiding each other with specialized biochemical tasks so as to maximize the chance that one of them will win the great race for the egg. See Baker, *Sperm Wars: The Science of Sex* (New York: HarperCollins, 1996).

Men themselves also compete in terms of "payload capacity." Humans and chimps have large testicles relative to body size; gorillas, small ones. Chimp and human lines diverged at least 6,000,000 years ago, and the first known patriarchal constraints on sex emerged about 5,000 years ago. During more than 99.9 percent of human development, then, the behavior that most societies today condemn and punish as promiscuity seems to have been the norm, and must still be intrinsic to human nature.

264 **church persuasion of cancer society:** Nicholas Wade, "Cancer Group in Controversy on Stem Cells," *New York Times*, 10 September 1999.

264 **Urban, Wilberforce, Bryan:** Pope Urban VIII, aka Maffeo Barberini, founder, in 1627, of the Collegium Urbanum, the Urban College of Propaganda (the first ad agency), was the pope who in 1633 explained to Galileo how the solar system works, at least the part within the orbit of Rome. Samuel Wilberforce, called "Soapy Sam" for his soapbox style, was the nineteenth-century Church of England point man against Darwinism, vastly out of his depth in public debates with Thomas Huxley. Bryan, three times a presidential candidate, was a major architect of Prohibition, and the prosecutor in the Scopes trial. His self-righteous ignorance, revealed under cross-examination by Clarence Darrow, made him the satirist H. L. Mencken's favorite ape.

274 **Phillips warns not to expect corporate ecosafety:** Carol Kaesuk Yoon, "What's Next for Biotech Crops? Questions," *New York Times*, 19 December 2000.

Selected Bibliography

Anders, George. *Health Against Wealth: HMOs and the Breakdown of Medical Trust*. New York: Houghton Mifflin, 1996.

Appleyard, Bryan. *Brave New Worlds: Staying Human in the Genetic Future*. New York: Viking Penguin, 1998.

Baer, Ellen Davidson, and Claire M. Fagin, eds. *Abandonment of the Patient: The Impact of Profit-Driven Health Care on the Public*. New York: Springer, 1996.

Bernstein, Peter L. *Against the Gods: The Remarkable Story of Risk*. New York: John Wiley, 1996.

Bogdanich, Walt. *The Great White Lie: How America's Hospitals Betray Our Trust and Endanger Our Lives*. New York: Simon & Schuster, 1991.

Callahan, Daniel. *False Hopes: Removing the Obstacles to a Sustainable, Affordable Medicine*. New York: Simon & Schuster, 1998.

Carlson, Rick J. *The End of Medicine*. New York: Basic Books, 1975.

Churchill, Larry. *Self Interest and Universal Health Care: Why Well-Insured Americans Should Support Coverage for Everyone*. Cambridge, Mass.: Harvard University Press, 1994.

Dawkins, Kristin. *Gene Wars: The Politics of Biotechnology*. Open Media Pamphlet Series. New York: Seven Stories Press, 1997.

Fukuyama, Francis. *The End of History and the Last Man*. New York: William Morrow, 1993.

Glasser, Ronald J. "The Doctor Is Not In: On the Failure of Managed Care." *Harper's*, March 1998.

Golub, Edward S. *The Limits of Medicine: How Science Shapes Our Hope for the Cure*. Chicago: University of Chicago Press, 1997.

Gordon, James. *Manifesto for a New Medicine: Your Guide to Healing Partnerships and the Wise Use of Alternative Therapies*. New York: Perseus, 1997.

Grace, Eric. *Biotechnology Unzipped: Promises and Realities*. Washington, D.C.: Joseph Henry Press, 1997.

Gray, Bradford H. *The Profit Motive and Patient Care: The Changing Accountability of Doctors and Hospitals*. Cambridge, Mass.: 20th Century Fund/Harvard University Press, 1992.

Herzlinger, Regina E. *Market-Driven Health Care: Who Wins, Who Loses in the Transformation of America's Largest Service Industry*. New York: Perseus, 1999.

Hitchens, Christopher. "Bitter Medicine." *Vanity Fair*, August 1998.

Kaplan, Jonathan. *The Limits and Lies of Human Genetic Research*. London: Routledge, 2000.

Kass, Leon R., and James Q. Wilson. *The Ethics of Human Cloning*. Washington, D.C.: AEI Press, American Enterprise Institute for Public Policy Research, 1998.

Keller, Evelyn Fox. *The Century of the Gene*. Cambridge, Mass.: Harvard University Press, 2000.

Kleinke, J. D. *Bleeding Edge: The Business of Health Care in the New Century*. New York: Aspen Publishers, 1998.

Konner, Melvin. *Medicine at the Crossroads: The Crisis in Health Care*. New York: Pantheon, 1993.

Lutz, Sandy, Woodrin Grossman, and John Bigalke. *Med Inc.: How Consolidation Is Shaping Tomorrow's Health Care System*. San Francisco: Jossey-Bass, 1998.

Maranto, Gina. *Quest for Perfection: The Drive to Breed Better Human Beings*. New York: Scribner's, 1996.

McGee, Glenn. *The Perfect Baby: A Pragmatic Approach to Genetics*. Lanham, Md.: Rowman & Littlefield, 1997.

McHughen, Alan. *Pandora's Picnic Basket: The Potential and Haz-*

ards of Genetically Modified Foods. New York: Oxford University Press, 2000.

Milunsky, Aubrey. *Your Genetic Destiny: Know Your Genes and Save Your Life*. New York: Perseus, 2001.

Miringoff, Marque-Luisa. *The Social Costs of Genetic Welfare*. New Brunswick, N.J.: Rutgers University Press, 1991.

Nelkin, Dorothy, and Lawrence R. Tancredi. *Dangerous Diagnostics: The Social Power of Biological Information*. Chicago: University of Chicago Press, 1994.

O'Brien, Lawrence J. *Bad Medicine: How the American Medical Establishment Is Ruining Our Healthcare System*. Amherst, N.Y.: Prometheus Books, 1999.

Ornish, Dean. *Love and Survival: The Scientific Basis of the Healing Power of Intimacy*. New York: HarperCollins, 1998.

Palmer, Julie Gage. *The Ethics of Human Gene Therapy*. New York: Oxford University Press, 1997.

Pence, Gregory. *Who's Afraid of Human Cloning?* Lanham, Md.: Rowman & Littlefield, 1998.

Ridley, Matt. *Genome: The Autobiography of a Species in 23 Chapters*. New York: HarperCollins, 1999.

Rifkin, Jeremy. *The Biotech Century: Harnessing the Gene and Remaking the World*. New York: Jeremy Tarcher/Putnam's, 1998.

Robinson, James C. *The Corporate Practice of Medicine: Competition and Innovation in Health Care*. Milbank Series on Health and the Public, no. 1. Berkeley, Calif.: University of California Press, 1999.

Rose, Steven. *Lifelines: Biology Beyond Determinism*. Oxford/New York: Oxford University Press, 1997.

Sagan, Leonard A. *The Health of Nations: True Causes of Sickness and Well-Being*. New York: Basic Books, 1987.

Schwartz, William B. *Life Without Disease: The Pursuit of Medical Utopia*. Berkeley: University of California Press, 1998.

Silver, Lee. *Remaking Eden: How Genetic Engineering and Cloning*

Will Transform the American Family. New York: HarperCollins/Avon, 1998.

Starr, Paul. *The Logic of Health-Care Reform: Transforming American Medicine for the Better*. Knoxville, Tenn.: Whittle Books, 1992.

Wade, Nicholas. *Life Script: How the Human Genome Discoveries Will Transform Medicine and Enhance Your Health*. New York: Simon & Schuster, 2001.

Walters, LeRoy, and Julie Gage Palmer. *The Ethics of Human Gene Therapy*. New York: Oxford University Press, 1996.

Wyke, Alexandra. *21st-Century Miracle Medicine*. New York: Plenum Press, 1997.

Index